THE PSYCHOTHERAPIST AND THE PROFESSIONAL COMPLAINT

THE SHADOW SIDE OF THERAPY

To my mother
Adah Sachs

To David, my husband
Valerie Sinason

EDITED BY ADAH SACHS AND VALERIE SINASON

THE PSYCHOTHERAPIST AND THE PROFESSIONAL COMPLAINT

THE SHADOW SIDE OF THERAPY

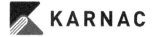 KARNAC

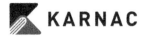

First published in 2023 by Karnac Books, an imprint of Confer Ltd.

www.confer.uk.com

Registered office:
Brody House, Strype Street, London E1 7LQ

1 3 5 7 9 10 8 6 4 2

Chapter 7 contains material from 'Serving two masters; a patient, a therapist,
and an allegation of sexual abuse' in Chapter 8 by Leslie Ironside, pp. 95–120,
in *Memory in Dispute*, edited by Valerie Sinason, Copyright © 1998 by Karnac Books.
Reproduced by permission of Taylor & Francis Group.

British Library Cataloguing in Publication Data
A catalogue record for this book is available from the British Library.

ISBN: 978-1-913494-61-2 (paperback)
ISBN: 978-1-913494-62-9 (ebook)

Typeset by Bespoke Publishing Ltd
Printed in the UK

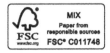

CONTENTS

ABOUT THE AUTHORS

Rajnish Attavar MD has been a Consultant Psychiatrist at Hertfordshire Partnership University NHS Foundation Trust since 2007, and works in Buckinghamshire. He was the clinical service director for Southern Health NHS Foundation Trust (Buckinghamshire and Oxfordshire) and has supported his organization in conducting Root Cause Investigations when needed. Dr. Attavar has a special interest in intellectual disability and psychotherapy, and is a training programme director for Thames Valley Deanery in intellectual disability. He is actively involved in research and teaching.

Richard Bagnall-Oakeley is an integrative psychotherapist (UKCP registered) and clinical supervisor, working with children, adolescents and adults in various settings in London. He was a founder member of the Psychotherapy and Counselling Union and served as Chair and then General Secretary of the union from 2017 to 2020. Before he became a therapist, Richard worked on adventure playgrounds with marginalized children and young people and was involved in grassroots activism with anti-capitalist and environmental groups. These experiences continue to inform his ethos of therapy as a playful, creative and anti-authoritarian endeavour.

Kay Beaumont is a retired social worker having worked for more than 40 years in many settings including adoption, mental health, learning disabilities, probation and as a guardian *ad litem*. She was a commissioner of forensic mental health services and a senior manager in an NHS mental health trust. She joined various Department of Health Groups including the Mansell Committee which reported on services for people with a learning disability and challenging behaviour. Her role has always included teaching, particularly inter-agency training with various clinicians as well as police officers. She has worked with both survivors of sexual abuse and sex offenders. Since retiring she has helped set up a service to support serious offenders with a diagnosis of personality disorder leaving prison or hospital. She is currently a panel member in a youth offending service.

Andrew Campbell-Tiech KC practises in London. He also sits as a Recorder in civil and criminal cases.

Philip Cox (DPsych) is an HCPC registered Chartered Psychologist, BPS Division of Counselling Psychology co-Vice Chair, BPS Psychotherapy Section past-Chair and BACP (Snr Accred) member, with over 25 years of clinical experience in multiple services. Phil is a founding member of the Psychotherapy & Counselling Union. His research publications, conference presentations and workshops focus on unintended harm within psychotherapy, and how to support people deemed to have misjudged the delicate balance between good and seemingly less helpful practice. Phil is a passionate advocate for social activism and supporting marginalised groups, which includes psychologists and psychotherapists who experience difficulties. Phil's philosophy is that by supporting therapists we support clients.

Emerald Davis is an Afro-Caribbean woman born in Guyana, who came to the UK at the age of nineteen. She trained as a nurse, becoming a psychiatric nurse, a midwife and a sister. She then found her lasting home in becoming an attachment-based psychoanalytic psychotherapist. As a therapist, she has focused on dissociation, disability and race. Emerald served as vice-Chair of the Bowlby Centre for eight years, and as Chair for further four years. She now has a small private practice in south London, as a training psychotherapist and supervisor.

Fiona Farley trained at The Royal Scottish Academy of Music and Drama and subsequently led a theatrical career for 25 years as an actor and an agent. This included co-founding 'Acting Associates', a cooperative actors' agency in London. In 2009 she obtained a Master's degree in art psychotherapy. She worked in Brighton and Sussex University Hospital with staff dealing with bereavement and Trauma; ran art-therapy workshops at Goodmayes Hospital in-patients wards, and was part of the psychotherapy team at PACE, an LGBTQ support service. She now lives in Edinburgh and is working in private practice, specializing in trauma and early childhood abuse. She has always felt that her acting experience enables her to feel herself into the life of another, which enriches her as a therapist.

Leslie Ironside (PhD) completed his training as a Child and Adolescent Psychotherapist in 1989 and his doctorate (on working with traumatized children) in 2001. Prior to this he worked as a teacher with emotionally disturbed children. From 1995 to 2004 he was a consultant psychotherapist in the NHS, while developing the Centre for Emotional Development as part of his private practice. He is currently the director of the Centre. Dr Ironside has a specialist interest in the field of fostering and adoption and has published a number of papers in this field. He is registered by Ofsted as an Adoption Support Agency rated 'outstanding'.

Professor Brett Kahr is Senior Fellow at the Tavistock Institute of Medical Psychology in London and, also, Visiting Professor of Psychoanalysis and Mental Health at Regent's University London. Additionally, he is Honorary Director of Research at Freud Museum London, as well as Chair of the Scholars Committee of the British Psychoanalytic Council. A Consultant Psychotherapist at The Balint

Consultancy, he works with individuals and couples in Central London. He is the author of 16 books and series editor of over 75 further titles. His most recent solo-authored book is entitled *Freud's Pandemics: Surviving Global War, Spanish Flu, and the Nazis*.

Sasha Kaplin trained in social work and spent years working in an NHS mental health crisis house for women. Through those years she was 'out' about being polyamorous, kinky and Jewish – the personal was political. Sasha also trained in systemic therapy and pursued a UKCP Integrative training. A battlesome exit from her training radicalized her perspective of therapy organizations, including the hegemony of registering bodies, and created a traumatized dissident. Her health deteriorated and she copes with disability. Her connection with Spiral, the Independent Practitioners Network and Pink Therapy sustained and helped her. Sasha puts her casework skills to use as a wounded activist healer and is PCU's Member Support Coordinator.

Anne Kearns DPsych (Prof) trained in psychoanalytic psychotherapy in the US and in Transactional Analysis and Gestalt psychotherapy in London at the Metanoia Institute, where she taught on their Masters and Doctoral programmes. Her doctoral project was entitled 'Professional Development and Informed Practice in the Area of Ethical Complaints' (Middlesex University 2007). She is the author of *The Seven Deadly Sins?* (Karnac, 2005) and *The Mirror Crack'd* (Karnac, 2011). Anne lives in south-west France and continues to work as a supervisor and expert witness and to support practitioners through the process of being complained against.

Dr Romanie Nedergaard-Couchman MD, MRCPsych is a Consultant Psychiatrist, specializing in working with people with learning disabilities and autism. Originally from the Netherlands, she completed her medical training in Amsterdam, the Netherlands, and her psychiatry specialty training in Oxfordshire. She has a broad experience in working with adults, children, older people, people with learning disabilities and autism, and a special interest in psychotherapy. She lives with her two young children and Corgi dog and loves spending time with them, travelling, practising yoga and being outdoors, ideally all together.

Julie Norris is a partner in the regulatory team at Kingsley Napley LLP. She advises professionals on regulatory compliance, investigations, adjudication, enforcement and prosecutions. In the health and social care sector, Julie advises doctors and talking therapy professionals facing disciplinary allegations. Julie is a member of the Professional Regulation Committee of the Law Society, the Professional Ethics Committee of the IBA and contributor to Thomson Reuters Practical Law Practice Compliance and Management.

Adah Sachs (PhD) is an attachment-based psychoanalytic psychotherapist and a training supervisor at the Bowlby Centre. She has worked for decades with adults and adolescents in psychiatric care, was a consultant psychotherapist at the Clinic for Dissociative Studies and is now retired from heading the NHS Psychotherapy Service for the London borough of Redbridge. Her main theoretical contribution is outlining subcategories of disorganized attachment, with links to trauma-based mental disorders. She writes, lectures and supervises worldwide on attachment and dissociation and is a fellow of the International Society for the Study of Trauma and Dissociation (ISSTD).

Valerie Sinason (PhD) is a poet, writer, child and adolescent psychoanalytic psychotherapist (retired) and adult psychoanalyst. She has specialized in trauma and disability for 40 years. She is a widely published writer and lectures nationally and internationally. Founder and Patron for the Clinic for Dissociative Studies UK, President of the Institute for Psychotherapy and Disability, she is on the Board of the International Society for the Study of Trauma and Dissociation (ISSTD). She received the ISSTD 2017 Lifetime Achievement Award and the British Psychoanalytic Council Innovation Excellence award in 2022. She has just published her first novel, *The Orpheus Project*.

Philip Stokoe (F.Inst.Psychoanal) is a Psychoanalyst in private practice working with adults and couples, and an Organizational Consultant, providing consultation to a wide range of organizations. He worked in the Adult Department of the Tavistock & Portman NHS Foundation Trust between 1994 and 2012, and was the Clinical Director from 2007. He is a member of the European Psychoanalytic Federation Forum on Institutional Matters, which studies the nature of psychoanalytic institutions. His book, *The Curiosity Drive: Our Need for Inquisitive Thinking*, was published in November 2020 and short-listed for the Gradiva® Award for Best Psychoanalytic Book in 2021.

ACKNOWLEDGEMENTS

Our thanks go to the patients who challenged and educated us; to the colleagues who supported us; to Karnac Books (especially Christina and Liz) for the enthusiastic encouragement at every stage; and to our authors for their willingness to think publicly about professional complaints.

As ever, our deepest thanks go to our families, for their hand-holding and love while we navigated the minefield, keeping our minds intact and evolving.

A NOTE FROM THE EDITORS

Adah Sachs and Valerie Sinason

This book was born out of complaints both editors went through (and were acquitted of). It took several years for the pain and shame to develop into a greater understanding of the dangers facing the therapeutic enterprise for all parties concerned. We hope this book will aid all members of our profession and inspire further thinking and change.

Two notes on language:

1. 'Psychotherapist' is used in this book as a global term for all mental health clinicians.
2. 'Patient' and 'client' are used interchangeably throughout the book.

INTRODUCTION
by Adah Sachs and Valerie Sinason

The psychotherapist and the professional complaint

Do you know anyone who has received a professional complaint? Maybe not. Or maybe you just don't know that they have. People don't tend to share such experiences.

Have you ever received a complaint? You would know, of course; but perhaps most of your colleagues never knew. Fear and shame silence such conversations.

This book aims to shed light on this shadowy topic and explore the practicalities, meanings, benefits and harms of the professional complaint. It looks at the historical development of the relationship between the professional and the patient. It compares different types of complaints – from the vexatious to the criminal, from the personal to the institutional, and the roles played in this process by the professional accrediting bodies, the NHS, a professional union, the legal system and the conscious and unconscious ethics of the profession. In particular, we explore the professional complaint through the experiences and thoughts of professionals who have been involved with the complaint process and were willing to contribute to the thinking about it: psychiatrists, advocates, scholars, counsellors, lawyers, psychologists, social workers, psychotherapists, psychoanalysts and activists.

Psychotherapy, in all its many forms, offers a relational framework in which entrenched pain and dysfunction can be shared, made sense of, lose their toxicity and hopefully be transformed into the live materials that build and enrich the Self. Undoing years of psychological hurts requires complex understanding and skill, and the training undertaken by psychotherapists is therefore demanding and lengthy.

All psychotherapy trainings include learning of theory, technique and practice; and they also include intensive psychotherapy for the trainee. As all people, clinicians have their own characterological weaknesses, life crises, vulnerabilities, pain, immaturities and blindness; and a crucial part of the ability to help others comes through recognizing one's own frailties and experiencing the process of their gradual transformation. This does not, of course, provide perfection: the negative aspect of the therapist's 'frailties' is that he or she is inevitably liable, at times, to be blindsided by them. The positive aspect is that character flaws, where recognized and processed, form the basis for the therapist's understanding and empathy, as well as their confidence – born from personal experience – that a level of transformation is possible.

Therapists, collectively, are also responsible for continually expanding their personal knowledge and the knowledge of the psychotherapy field. For this reason, further to their qualifying training, therapists are also required to undertake continuing professional development (CPD), and receive some form of supervision. They are also encouraged to write, publish, research and lecture. Subsequently, human difficulties which have not previously been understood or recognized gradually find their place in the expanding scope of the field. Forensic psychotherapy, disability therapy, antenatal mental health, addiction, complex trauma therapy and the treatment of dissociative disorders – to name but a few – are all quite new. Until recently, people with these and other minority needs were neither recognized nor treated, or were treated with a crass lack of understanding. While sticking to what we already know is easier and may feel 'safer', excluding whole groups of people from care can hardly be ethical. Expanding our scope of practice, however, inevitably increases the risks of 'getting it wrong'. This is one of the many ethical conundrums of the profession; and as we must assume that the risk of misstep, mistake and even wrongdoing is forever present in our work, the obvious question is: where something has gone wrong, what could put it right?

In most cases, problems which occur between patient/client and their therapist get resolved within the therapy. Indeed, the ability to do so is an important area of therapy, and a satisfying resolution is a significant therapeutic achievement. But when a problem cannot be put right by the process of therapy itself, we still need to respond to what the patient needs or indeed wants when they feel wronged by their therapist. Making a complaint against the therapist allows a third party (normally an ethics committee or the accrediting body of the therapist) to step in and decide whether – and to what extent – the therapist has done wrong, and what sanctions – if any – should follow as a result.

The complaint process allows the patient a recourse; it allows the therapist to respond, explain their line of thinking and recognize mistakes; it brings wrongdoing to light and maintains professional standards. However, it is not without a cost, and it has the potential to seriously harm all the people involved. For the patient, it carries the risk that their complaint may be dismissed, leaving them more hurt and feeling even less understood than before. For the therapist, it is an incredibly harsh ordeal which can last many months. While it goes on, the therapist may be barred from seeing other patients (who get hurt as innocent bystanders), and it can harm the therapist's reputation and career even if it later transpires that they had done no wrong.

Furthermore, almost invariably, the therapy relationship ends up irreparably broken following a complaint. Once this complex entity, *The Complaint*, has entered the space between patient and therapist it almost always destroys that space.

Most patients make a complaint because they feel hurt, angry and wronged, and they want to force their therapist to do better by punishing him or her for poor form. Most patients do not want the therapy to end, or they would have just left; they want the therapist to improve. Having to endure months of waiting, at the end of which the therapist may or may not have been punished but the therapy was destroyed and came to an end (rather than improved) can feel like being cheated: the therapist (even if punished) got away from the patient, not changed for the better. The patient was abandoned, not treated better.

Similar (if not quite as high-stake) dynamics can be seen in complaints made against therapists by their employers, professional organizations or colleagues.

There is a very hard-to-maintain balance in the complaint option: on the one hand, it runs the risk of crippling the psychotherapy relationship by forcing it into a culture of 'defensive practice'. On the other hand, we must have a way to protect against the predatory and otherwise unethical clinician. For all its potential damage, it is hard to see how we could manage without having a process which allows wrongs to be exposed and dealt with.

It matters, and it is deeply therapeutic, that wrongs be put right. It also matters that the process of 'putting right' is not an invitation for revenge and destruction of what matters the most. Like alchemy, the process of therapy aims to transform the base, twisted metals of harsh experiences and suffering into the gold nuggets which build the Self. It also requires a careful watch, so that the hard-earned gold not be turned into the base metals of destruction. It is our hope that our shared thinking in the following pages will help us to find the way.

PART I

CLINICAL PERSPECTIVE

CHAPTER I

The psychotherapist, the profession and the professional complaint

Adah Sachs

This paper was born out of a personal experience: I received a complaint. It was resolved in my favour, so one could say that it ended well (for me), but it had a shocking beginning and a pretty awful middle, and it caused the greatest confusion of my professional life to date. It also made me think in much more depth about the shadow side of the relationship between patient and therapist, where the deep attunement, attention and affection that characterize the relationship can suddenly turn dysfunctional and dangerous.

Writing these words brought back to memory the only time I was physically hit by a patient. She was a long-stay inpatient, and I went to her room to pick her up for her session as I did every Tuesday and Thursday at 11.00 a.m. On that day, however, I found her door closed and very loud music blaring from inside the room. I knocked on the door, but the music was too loud for her to hear it. I opened the door a crack: she stood at the far end of the room, her back to me, looking out of the window. I called her name, but my voice was drowned by the music. Walking slowly in, I reached for the volume dial and turned it down. Quick as a flash, she turned round and kicked me. We both froze.

That kick was a raw complaint. It said, quite rightly, that I had no right to touch her radio. That I trampled over her privacy. That I forcefully took away her music instead of listening to it and thinking about it. That I was a bad therapist and a scary person. A moment of misattunement, impatience and acting out (mine) was met by a moment of indignant and fearful rage and acting out (hers), derailing our relationship in seconds into a dysfunctional exchange. And we froze, shocked by the intensity of negative affects and by the loss of our shared language.

Thankfully, it did not take long for attunement and thinking to return. I apologized, and the work continued. In fact, that breakdown moment ended up being pivotal to the therapy.

In this chapter, however, I examine the process of a 'real', formal complaint (rather than a kick), focusing particularly on its problematic, *unintended* consequences.

I should note here that this subject has not previously been an area of interest to me. Indeed, prior to receiving one, I had hardly given a thought to professional complaints: in my mind, they were vaguely connected to unethical, predatorial or plain bad therapists – issues that, naively, I did not consider to have any relevance to me. I also confess to having a deep impatience towards the bureaucratic, administrative elements of life, and the words 'complaint procedures' seemed to fall in that very dull category. Well, I no longer think so.

Finding myself on the receiving end of a formal complaint was not dull. It was shocking. For a time, I couldn't think at all, such was the impact of it. It was also quite gripping, in a horrifying, all-consuming kind of way: the initial shock was followed by months where I could hardly think about anything else. Ultimately, though, it was an eye-opener. An eye-opener about the shadow side of our relationship with our patients: how close to the surface are the vulnerability, aggression and fear in each of us and between us (Winnicott, 1949). An eye-opener about the limitations of my personal robustness, and the limitations of *our collective professional robustness*. And perhaps an eye-opener to some of the personality traits common in therapists that contribute to our lack of robustness as a group.

These thoughts and realizations made me choose to end this paper not at the 'happy end' point where the complaint against me was dismissed, but with a discussion about the conscious and unconscious relationship between the psychotherapist, the profession and the professional complaint.

A case study: the complaint I received

A few years ago, following decades of intense clinical work, I decided that the time had come for me to take a sabbatical year. I gave my patients one year notice of my plan and settled into the process of endings. As was to be expected, this was not easy; but eventually there was a resolution and a proper ending with each of my patients. All except one.

This one patient, who I will call John, was unable to accept my 'bailing out on him'. He raged, suffered, became suicidal, hated me for my selfishness, betrayal, cruelty and heartlessness, hated himself for his dependence and neediness and denigrated both of us. After several months of suffering (both his and mine), he met a therapist whom he liked and told me that as the new therapist was 'so much better than me' he wanted to start working with him immediately and was not going to wait for the end of our agreed time.

I believe my response was a mistake, probably driven by my exhaustion after being emotionally battered for months: I accepted his announcement of a unilateral, early ending of our work, and said I was impressed by his taking charge of his own process, rather than feeling beholden to my timetable. While I tried to convince myself that my response was 'enabling', I did know that it was not entirely so. Congratulating him on his independent choice had robbed him of the opportunity to 'slam the door in my face', and I'm afraid that, being a sensitive person, he may have been quite aware that my 'positive' acceptance of his choice reflected my (not so positive) longing to end these punishing sessions as soon as possible.

But these are just my own thoughts. I have not seen John again since his announcement of his immediate ending, and the day after his departure I was informed by his new therapist that John wanted no contact with me whatsoever.

On my return to the UK at the end of my sabbatical, I was greeted by a hefty, special delivery envelope containing a fifty-page *Professional Complaint* document. Thirty-five pages were written by John. The other fifteen were entitled 'a witness statement', written by John's new therapist.

The contents of the complaint were not about the poor quality of my work or about my selfishness, lack of sensitivity or heartlessness (all of which I could have understood, given our difficult ending). The complaint consisted of detailed descriptions of abuse and torture. John stated that, throughout the years of his work with me, I had repeatedly punished him for his thoughts and behaviours, and my punishments were cruel and terrifying: he said that I had often locked him up overnight in my consulting room, naked and alone, with no heating in the empty building; that on several occasions I had sent him naked into the street at the end of a session; that I had inserted various objects into his anus; tried to strangle him with a nylon cord around his neck; attempted to drown him by pushing his head under water in the WC's basin; and when he didn't 'work hard enough' in therapy, I forced his hands on to a lit stove. These, and many similar items, filled thirty-five single-spaced pages. The 'witness statement' contained a shorter version of some of the events already described in John's complaint.

I was dumbstruck.

My first thought, when I was able to think again, was relief that it was not a complaint about my rather scanty record-keeping. This one was so extreme that it was obviously material for therapy, not for an accrediting body evaluation. The intense vulnerability he described (being naked and alone in the cold, desperately needing protection and warmth, yet staying in my consulting room overnight), the torment I had caused him by fire and water, the feeling – terror – that I was 'killing him' and his anguished cry for something or someone to stop me (from leaving? from locking him *out of* the consulting room?) all needed to be thoughtfully and compassionately disentangled and linked to his inner reality, so that his outer reality could make sense.

I was not, however, asked to write a therapeutic case study, or to speak to John. I was required to 'respond to each item'. What could I possibly say to a committee about any of these items? Was I expected to state that none of these were true? Surely no one would possibly think they were!

But my next thought was, could anyone, when hearing such a ghastly tale, actually suspect me? Clearly, John's new therapist had not questioned his claims about my abuse of him, he even named himself a 'witness' to the events described, as if he had actually been there and knew them to be true. How many other professionals may think so?

Moreover, what would be my own reaction to a therapist accused of such crimes, even if I knew the therapist and generally thought well of them? Would I think it was obviously phantasy material or a deliberate revenge, or would I wonder if there was perhaps something in it? Accounts of hard-to-believe abuse were not infrequently proven to be true (Middleton, 2013; Middleton et al, 2018; Salter, 2013); and through decades of my own work with abuse victims I knew that the people committing such crimes may not 'look like abusers'. Assuming my close colleagues shared similar experience and views to my own, why would they not suspect me?

As well as the shock at considering that my innocence (and indeed sanity) were questioned, I also found myself in a fundamental cognitive and moral dilemma: how could I possibly say – or even think – the words 'this is mad, no one will ever believe you'? These were the very words that abusers told their victims, in order to silence them. The thought of myself silencing a person by dismissing his account as 'outlandish, therefore untrue' went against the grain of my thinking, and anything I had ever practised, written and taught (e.g. Middleton et al, 2018; Sachs 2007, 2011, 2013, 2017).

Nevertheless, John was not telling the truth. Unlike other situations where I heard a patient's accounts of his or her traumatic history (including John's own accounts of his childhood abuse), in this case I had the unusual 'luxury' of certainty about the facts: I knew that the crimes he described had not been committed. His complaint may have described an internal experience, a memory or his rage at me and his wish for revenge, but it was not an account of my actions. To my mortification, I found myself wondering if some of his accounts of his childhood abuse may not have been true either, a question which returned me to my cognitive and moral dilemma.

Guilty until proven innocent

Back at my desk, I was required to respond to each item, to prove my innocence. Given the document's length, this took me several days. Meanwhile, my accrediting body was seeking a suitable investigating officer for this complaint. The task of an investigating officer is to collect all relevant material supplied by both sides, read it and make a recommendation as to whether or not there was a case to answer. An investigating officer must have sufficient expertise in the main areas of the complaint and be agreed to by both sides. Given the complexities of the case, the search for a suitable person took several stressful months. There was nothing for it but waiting.

Chinese whispers

Meanwhile, in our not-so-large professional world, the story of this complaint started to spread during the months of waiting. Two of my supervisees who were in therapy with John's new therapist cancelled their work with me. A colleague of mine sent me a cryptic message about having a problem with being in the same meeting with me because of potential conflict with a client of hers. Some of my colleagues in the US had heard about it and asked me if the story was true; and one of them said she read it on a group email from a colleague of John's therapist. I felt my paranoia rising: what did my colleagues think of me? Would anyone ever trust me again? Should I step down from a board of directors I was serving on, so as not to contaminate the reputation of the organization with a pending complaint of this nature? I was due to give a paper at an international conference and wondered how I could face meeting people. I felt a crushing weight of shame for being even associated with such a complaint; fear of losing all my friends and colleagues, and anger for being put in such a position. It is remarkable how easy it is to tarnish – perhaps permanently – a therapist's name, and potentially destroy their career. I was being punished for no crime and was to remain guilty until proven innocent.

The sting

Just when a suitable investigating officer was finally found and the process appeared to be moving forward, I was informed that John and his therapist had dropped the complaint. Had they realized that it was not likely to go in John's favour? Was John becoming too distressed by the complaint he'd made several months earlier when he was upset, now it was becoming more 'real' as he was required to meet with the investigating officer and repeat words that, somewhere in his mind, he must have known were untrue? Be that as it may, it meant that this complaint could not ever be really closed. Were John and his therapist devious enough to choose this course of action deliberately, so as to keep me forever suspected?

I made a request for the investigation to continue until a conclusion was reached but was told that there was no provision for such course of action: dropping a complaint was the prerogative of the person making it. My accrediting body regulators, the relevant ethics committee, the organization within which I saw John for several years were all terribly sympathetic, but there didn't seem to be any way to resolve the situation.

A nasty complaint, which circulates for a few months while 'confidentially' shared with colleagues and friends and is then simply dropped with no formal resolution can cause terrible damage, and there was apparently no remedy for it. 'Guilty until proven innocent' was to become my permanent professional status. And as in the absence of a complaint innocence could not be proven, I was left with 'guilty'. It felt as though I had fallen off the edge.

Resolution

After some weeks of avoiding meeting people and becoming increasingly distraught, I realized that I must come out my cave and speak to my friends and colleagues in the hope of gaining some wisdom, advice and emotional support. I steeled myself and with great trepidation started to tell my colleagues: I've had a complaint, and I have no idea what to do. To my surprise, people were very sympathetic. Some of them started to tell me about complaints they had had but never talked about. When I told them what it was about (excluding the participants' identities) they were flabbergasted at first and then supportive. They reminded me that I was a good person, and that they couldn't possibly believe that I had actually tried to murder a patient. When I confessed my dread of going to the conference I was due to speak at, some immediately offered to come with me. Not going alone felt less scary.

I informed the board of directors I was serving on of my situation and asked whether I should step down. After discussion, the board's reply was an unequivocal 'no'. There was no decision against me, no evidence was brought forward, and I had no previous 'form'. All that was on the table were unsupported accusations and rumours. Rumours don't count, I was told, only evidence. Furthermore, they emphasized that damaging rumours were illegal and encouraged me to get legal advice.

I found a lawyer, who, after reading the documents made several points:
   a. Contrary to his statement, John's therapist was not a witness to any of the events he described, because he wasn't there. Presumably, he had heard these accounts from John and believed him, but this was hearsay, not independently known facts and certainly not evidence.
   b. The therapist was breaking the law: spreading accusations with no evidence was slanderous and libellous.
   c. John, too, was breaking the law if he was knowingly making a false claim against me.

The lawyer sent a letter to this effect to John's therapist, instructing him to 'cease and desist', and to put everyone he had 'shared' the story with on notice that they, too, may be deemed slanderous and libellous.

She also advised me that I had sufficient grounds to go back to my accrediting body and state that by not concluding the investigation, they were exposing me to slander and libel and may be held responsible for the outcome. Within a few days the investigation reopened, and a few days later, in the absence of any response from John or his therapist, it closed with a 'no case to answer' conclusion.

Afterward: why?

This question continued to haunt me for years. Why did John do it? And even more surprising, why did his therapist? I really wish I knew, but having had no contact with either of them since my work with John ended, all I can offer here are my own thoughts and, not wishing to overindulge in speculation, I will keep this short.

I could think of John's action in a similar way to the patient who kicked me: I – insensitively – touched a nerve, and received a knee-jerk reaction (literally, from the first patient). However, while telling his new therapist how much torture I've inflicted on him may have been an unmitigated outpouring of hurt and rage, John went far further than a knee-jerk: filling in the complaint forms, writing – and signing for the truthfulness of – thirty-five pages of detailed description and keeping the process going for several months required tenacity of purpose over time. The thought of a patient motivated by a persistent destructive wish towards his therapist is a chilling one, but I now think that it is one which must be held in mind as a possibility.

The motivation for John's therapist's actions is even less clear to me. First, he must have realized that John was very upset and needed a listening ear. With this in mind, it would have made sense for him to consider John's accusations on many (psychological) levels prior to engaging in supporting the concrete act of launching a complaint. Indeed, had he really believed John's account of horrific abuse done by me and was truly concerned about the safety of John and potentially any of my other patients (or of other members of the public, for that matter), he should have gone to the police, not to an ethics committee. Attempting to murder your patient is not a breach of ethics. It's an extremely serious crime.

On the other hand, if he did not really believe John and was not actually worried, did he make a gratuitous complaint simply to please John, or for cementing their bond? Supporting a client in making claims that were – in the external world – false, is wrong on every count: it is a lie; it attacks an innocent person, and it is clinically harmful. While it may create a temporary feeling of trust or bonding with the patient, it could ultimately only lead to disappointment and to clinical deterioration due to the disappointment, lies and the confusion between inside and outside reality.

John's therapist is a known professional and a bright man. I could hardly think he would have missed these considerations. Perhaps being in the role of a 'replacement therapist' to a traumatized and needy patient had evoked a deep wish in him to be John's saviour. While such sentiments are not uncommon, they rarely reach such proportions as these.

But let's remember, these are merely my speculations. I don't know why they decided to make the complaint, or what was the impact on John.

Notes on weaknesses in the current complaint procedures

This complaint had to be concluded not by considering its *central* points (the alleged abuse of a patient) but through an intervention of a lawyer who pointed out *secondary* breaches of the law (slander). It was thus not a fully satisfactory resolution, but it was the only way to proceed because the existing procedures had no means to resolve this situation or indeed this type of complaint. I'd like to highlight a few specific points which, I believe, are behind the inability of the system to manage some complaints:

Scope

Professional complaint procedures are intended for investigating *ethical breaches*. Unlike statutory bodies, professional accrediting bodies do not have the means (or authority) to investigate whether or not an act had actually been committed, or for searching for evidence. Where the alleged acts are disputed or denied, especially when these acts are of a criminal nature (like in the case I have described), an impasse is inevitable because the critical question is not whether an act was *ethical*, but whether or not it *had actually happened*, a question the complaint process has no way to answer.

Defining the scope (and the limits) of what a professional complaint can cover is essential. Excluding at the outset complaints which are outside the scope of ethical consideration (for example, criminal allegations) and directing them to appropriate investigators (the police, social services, and so on) seems like a realistic, practical solution.

Clarity

Complaint procedures do not, at present, differentiate between complaints made by a patient, a colleague or an institution, applying the same rules to all of them (see more under 'balance'). They also do not make a distinction between the roles of a witness, an advocate and a therapist, which I argue are mutually exclusive:

A **witness** is a person who knows what had happened, because they were there at the time and had witnessed the relevant events. The witness must be accurate, objective and truthful.

An **advocate** is a person who is explicitly on the patient's side. The advocate does not claim neutrality and does not need to have been there when the events happened. Their role is to help the patient understand and/or express him or herself fully, that is, be a bridge between a vulnerable person and the world.

A **therapist**, conversely, is almost never a witness to the patient's history (because he or she were not there when it happened). A therapist account is thus not a testimony of facts. It is, by definition, a hearsay. The therapist is also not an advocate: his or her role is to help patients understand themselves better and find their own truth.

These differentiations are critically important, and mixing these roles is bound to cause mistakes and injustice, as well as harming the therapy itself. If a patient relies on the advocacy (support) or testament (statement of facts) of their therapist, it will inevitably impact on what the patient says to their therapist, thus undermining the objectivity of the testament and harming the therapy.

Balance

It appears to me that the central flaw in the existing procedure is that a complaint is unevenly balanced in favour of the one making it.

1. The balance of harm

A professional complaint damages the reputation of the therapist and casts doubt on his or her capability or moral ground even if it is later dismissed. It can cause loss of earnings (if the therapist is prevented from practising while being investigated) and serious damage to the therapist's future career. In other words, it acts as a punishment even where there was no misdeed. Conversely, there is no cost – financial or reputational – for making a vexatious complaint, even where it is later found to be baseless or completely false. This imbalance carries the risk for complaints being misused and weaponized (for example, by an angry or vindictive colleague or patient) rather than serving as a tool for improving professional standards.

2. The balance of the burden of proof

The burden of proof in a professional complaint is primarily on the accused, who must prove their innocence so as to be free to return to normal practice (including being eligible to renew their insurance cover and professional registration). The complainant is under no restrictions while the complaint is being processed and can even change their mind and drop the case at any point with impunity.

This is the opposite sensibility to that of the law, where one is deemed innocent until proven guilty, and the burden of proof is on the accuser.

3. The balance of legal responsibility in the clinical relationship

The lawyer I saw pointed out that John (in addition to his therapist) had also broken the law by making and signing a false statement. As a member of the public, she said, John was liable and could be sued. I have obviously not pursued this option because John had been my patient and I attributed his actions to his poor mental health. It does however, beg the question: should our professional code exempt our patients, present and past, from legal responsibility in relationship to their therapists? Should this be part of our contract, whether explicit or implicit?

Are all patients equal?

This is another thorny question. Differentiating between patients on grounds of their diagnosis screams of discrimination and has a harrowing history of mistreatment and cruelty. We are, thankfully, no longer allowed to discriminate against any patient (Nedergaard-Couchman and Attavar, see Chapter 10).

However, the persistently serious shortage of clinicians in some clinical areas (for example, psychosis, personality disorders, dissociative disorders) does amount to 'stealth discrimination', which is not based on prejudice but on risk, including an elevated risk of complaints (Sinason, see Chapter 5). Having spent most of my career in these areas (including carrying statutory responsibility for many of the patients), I know the cost of the lack of treatment for these highly vulnerable patient groups, but also how tough is the work for the too-few clinicians, who are necessarily exposed to greater professional risk because of the nature of the work. Our professional systems must not ignore the increased burden and subsequent needs of clinicians in these areas and, to paraphrase Winnicott (1973), support the therapists in supporting the patients.

Protective function

Our accrediting bodies have educational, accrediting and regulatory functions, the latter aimed at protecting the public. But as mentioned, they have no function of protecting the therapist against risks which are due to the nature of the therapist's work. Considering that we ourselves have created our various accrediting bodies, this is a curious omission.

The professional complaint: psychotherapists' unconscious view of themselves

Like all unconscious material, it can only be seen through the cracks of our conscious mind: through our 'curious omissions', contradictory choices, the gaps between what we do and what we think we meant. Looking at our attitudes towards ourselves in the context of our profession reveals many such contradictions, particularly regarding our own strength.

We are used to seeing signs in GP surgeries and hospitals, on buses and in public offices, reminding the public that 'anyone abusing our staff will be prosecuted'. But psychotherapists do not offer themselves any protection within the therapeutic relationship. It seems that we believe we need none, or perhaps deserve none.

Admitting (if only to ourselves or to a trusted supervisor) to being afraid, disgusted, annoyed or exhausted by a patient feels unprofessional and evokes embarrassment, guilt or both. Our unconscious view of ourselves appears to hold that we are inherently unaffected. Obviously, this doesn't match reality.

At the same time, we also shy away from the explicit acknowledgement of our professional strength, and the inherent imbalance of power within the therapeutic relationship. Many therapists don't like the word 'patient' as it suggests that one side is ill and the other healthy. Some schools of therapy go so far as rejecting altogether the notion of 'getting better' through therapy (and thus through the therapist), speaking about therapy as 'a shared journey', and stressing the equality of the participants in the journey in opposition to seeing the psychotherapist as a professional. Yet we were quick to undertake some of the most punitive (to ourselves) professional codes, aiming to ensure that therapists do not misuse their professional position, as though we deem ourselves inherently, dangerously, bad.

So, we are uncomfortable with accepting – and expressing – our weakness and need for protection, and we are also uncomfortable with stating our professionalism, learned skill, and the natural authority that comes with any skill. We must help without seeming to do so, and without seeming to have any needs or interests of our own. Somehow, we must not be fully human, because our strength may be harmful and our weakness unacceptable.

Perhaps this is a reflection of an unconscious guilt about the monumental privilege of our profession – that of being allowed into the psyche of another. Humbled by this privilege we may feel that we can ask for or deserve nothing more, and that we are never allowed to err in the slightest.

Or perhaps a kinder – and more hopeful – explanation to our unreasonable severity may be found elsewhere. Perhaps we are still in the midst of the quest to 'find ourselves' because, as a profession, we are still young, and youthfulness entails both over-confidence and under-confidence. Attempting maturity, we have created a variety of professional structures: long trainings, professional registration, ethical principles and provisions for protecting our patient's safety, including complaint procedures. We have not created a structure for protecting ourselves. Yet.

Perhaps this will come with further maturity.

CHAPTER 2

When healing is halted by fear

Fiona Farley

W e do our work with no witnesses, in small private rooms. This has been the tried and tested 'proven' way to create a safe environment for over a hundred years. Its primary intention is to provide a space that enables the healing to happen. We have been taught to respect the Therapeutic Frame (Bleger, 1967) by creating confidentiality, consistency and reliability for the client. However, defining the therapeutic relationship is difficult. One way is the term 'working alliance'. The alliance has been well defined by Bordin as 'the bond between the participants, the extent of their agreement on the goals of therapy, and the extent of their agreement on the task' (Bordin, 1979).

In my experience as an integrative arts psychotherapist, if a deep, trusting, intimate relationship can be built, the client is more likely to feel able to go to their dark places and access their innermost feelings. Whatever modality is being practised, an impressive body of research shows that the relationship is the core healing tool (Frank, 1979; Farber and Doolin, 2011; Kolden, Klein, Wang and Austin, 2011). As Rollo May (1969) puts it, 'it's the relationship that heals'.

> 'Fundamentally, if a psychotherapist can establish a relationship with someone who has lost the capacity for relationship, he or she has been retrieved in their relatedness with others. Thus they can begin to rejoin the family of man.' (Clarkson, 1993, p.24)

Most people would agree that good relationships are nurturing but they also produce conflict and misunderstanding. The only way any of us have to explore this in a relationship is to acknowledge to the other we do not like something that is happening. In other words, make a complaint.

I have often found complaints from clients extremely helpful; they have been useful for the work and taught me an enormous amount. I have worked with a client for six years who has a diagnosis of DID (Dissociative Identity Disorder). She has an Alter (they use the term Person) who appears when something I have said or done has been triggering or traumatizing for the system. She is fearless, intelligent, protective and very critical. I will sometimes receive a list of all the things I 'got wrong' in the previous session. These might be words I said that upset her (which I had no idea were triggers to past trauma). She has also pointed out when I have avoided emotional connection by challenging her intellectually. In the early days of working with this client I found it very challenging. It was humbling when I realized this person, who had suffered more than I could even imagine, had so much to teach me. Out of all the clients I have worked with over the years, she has had the biggest single influence in making me a better therapist.

The therapeutic relationship is unique, when successful it is truthful, caring and safe. It also contains a complete power imbalance. The client is encouraged to share their most vulnerable history, their shame, their hopes and dreams; whilst the therapist remains an enigma. We endeavour to bring an authenticity to this relationship, the client hopefully receives our compassion, is confident in our professional knowledge and experiences some of our personality, but the rule is 'no personal disclosures'.

In private practice the exchange of a fee for the therapist's time is often a significant redress of the power balance, but it can also introduce more doubt into the relationship. Clients can wonder if you are only there for the money and don't really care about them. It can even produce a transference of a sexual nature, when a client is 'buying time' with you. In a fascinating way, these intimacies and power dynamics come together to create a relationship that contains elements of every other relationship in that person's life. When the therapist is confident enough to work with the transference and countertransference (Freud, 1912/1959), it becomes a rich fertile environment of self-enquiry and psychotherapeutic healing. According to Klein:

'Such retrospective insight is based on one of the crucial findings of Freud, the transference situation, that is to say the fact that in a psycho-analysis the patient re-enacts in relation to the psycho-analyst earlier – and, I would add, even very early – situations and emotions. Therefore the relationship to the psycho-analyst at times bears, even in adults, very childlike features, such as over-dependence and the need to be guided, together with quite irrational distrust.' (Klein, 1997, p.247)

The neuroscientist Louis Cozolino suggests that,

'Later relationships and/or the working through and integration of childhood experiences is possible. Earned autonomy appears capable of interrupting the transmission of negative attachment patterns from one generation to the next. It is what we hope will happen through the process of psychotherapy' (Cozolino, 2006, p. 313).

Given the fact that we are often working with vulnerable and damaged people, this very hothouse of emotional ingredients can also produce enormous rage. When the client experiences a need to lash out at everything and every person who has ever hurt them, this can be transferred on to the therapist who has 'made them feel it'.

The only power the client has to express that rage is to 'punish' the therapist. This 'punishment' can take many forms in the therapy room. When worked with skilfully there is a rich vein of healing to be gained, however, sometimes the client choses to take their anger outside of the one to one relationship and makes a complaint against the therapist to some big, powerful governing body. What better way to have their pain and abuse seen and the 'perpetrator' punished, than by exposing the pain we have helped unleash to our 'parent' organization.

The following example shows how a small unconscious mishandling of an email can quickly explode into potentially catastrophic proportions.

My client was a 45-year-old white, heterosexual, female, presenting with relationship difficulties, intrusive thoughts and erratic mood swings. She had been diagnosed at 18 with BPD (borderline personality disorder) and saw an NHS psychiatrist once a year to discuss current medication. She had been hospitalized four or five times since her late teens after psychotic episodes.

We had worked together, with some breaks, for five years when she decided to end her therapy. I suggested we continue for a few sessions, working towards an ending, but after acknowledging the importance of our work together and what she would be taking away with her from it, she decided to end that day. There followed at various intervals, usually on a weekend, one-line texts saying 'hello' or 'I'm thinking of you'. I did not reply to any of these texts. I was aware that this client had grown up without a secure attachment and had a chaotic relationship with her partner. I suspected our therapeutic relationship had been the first experience of a healthy relationship and she was finding it difficult to let go of it. After eight months of receiving these occasional texts from her I received an email asking for a session. My private practice was full and it was four days before the Christmas holidays. I say this to put my response into contexts, not to excuse myself from any error. I replied with a short but truthful email, saying my practice was absolutely full just now and that I had nothing available until well into the New Year. I suggested she might want to consult another therapist and that I was happy to make some recommendations. The response I received was full of hurt and anger, followed by rage. She considered my reply to be lacking in professional care and informed me she was not only going to lodge a complaint with my professional body, the UKCP (UK Council for Psychotherapy) but also pursue me through the courts for compensation for professional misconduct.

I could have handled this better; in hindsight my email was rushed and without sufficient compassion. I do not however believe it was a case for a professional misconduct inquiry. So why was I so frightened? I immediately called my supervisor and my insurance company. My supervisor made herself available at short notice, she was very supportive of me and concerned for the client. I could also hear tension and slight anxiety in her voice. It is very possible that she was experiencing projective identification from me, coupled with her own fears of the potential threat to her own professional reputation.

> 'Projective identification describes the process whereby a client unconsciously conveys his/her feelings by "giving" the therapist an experience of how he/she feels, rather than by articulating. The therapist does not, cannot, actually feel the client's feelings but the client evokes similar feelings in the therapist.' (Mackewn, 1997, p. 95)

My professional liability insurance company were the most helpful at this time. I was transferred directly through to one of their lawyers, who said she couldn't see any grounds for misconduct but asked me to forward all the email correspondence and instructed me to contact her should it go any further. I felt instantly calmer, trusted and protected.

One of our biggest fears as therapists is having an official complaint made about us. We fear humiliation, loss of respect from our peers, loss of our ability to work, loss of the confidence of future clients and our reputation, but most of all personal doubt in our ability to do our job well. In the private world of the therapy room, there is only 'their word against ours', no outside evidence and no protection from a false claim of misconduct or abuse of power. All our years of training, our vocational desire to use our skills for healing, our membership of professional bodies, whose codes of conduct we study and adhere to, do nothing to protect us from the irrational, unsubstantiated claims of hurt and angry clients. This is because the client often actually believes the abuse took place, because they genuinely feel abused, powerless, judged and mistreated. In successful therapy, feelings brought back into the relationship and reflected on, can help the client see that their historical suffering is affecting their current relationships. Rupture and repair are at the heart of deepening every relationship, especially the therapeutic one.

There is evidence that not only does the repair of ruptures benefit the work, but that treatments in which there are ruptures that are repaired may be superior in effectiveness to treatments in which there are no known ruptures. Thus, the existence of ruptures may be seen as a good thing, as signifying that the therapist is doing his or her work, so long as the rupture gets repaired (Gelso, 2019, p.64).

This can be incredibly powerful work, using the therapeutic relationship to help the client out of historical patterns and into more peaceful, satisfying ways of relating. It can demonstrate a healthy relationship that survives difficulties. Often the client can internalize this model of relationship and begin to take it into their personal lives. However, when the therapist becomes frightened and the complaints procedure kicks in, the client may permanently lose the opportunity to continue the work they were doing.

In my opinion, the current way of handling complaints of this nature is ultimately punishing the most needy and damaged clients. I also wonder if the fact that our professional bodies are carrying out investigations into complaints is contributing to the problem. Possibly this is linked to the fact we are not a government regulated profession. Perhaps if there was an external body created for all complaints about psychotherapists and counsellors, our individual professional bodies could support us better. To gain membership of the UKCP I had to rigorously prove my fitness to practise. Each year, I am required to present an account of my continued professional training, the number of supervision hours I have per number of clients and the professional books and journals I have read or contributed to. Every five years I have an even more in-depth enquiry into my continued professional development and my current working practice. I would like a professional body that assumes innocence until proven otherwise by another organization. With the feeling of someone 'having my back' and believing in my professional decisions, I might be more likely to attempt to continue working with the aggrieved and troubled client.

Regarding the case I am writing about, a few weeks into that new year, having spent an anxious holiday waiting for her next move, I began to internally connect to how she might be feeling. I remembered our work together and how vulnerable she was. After some in-depth self-inquiry around my reasons, I decided to phone her to ask how she was doing. I could only do this when I found myself coming from a place of compassionate, professional care. I also wanted to take control of the situation rather than living with the expectation of impending disaster. She was friendly and dismissive of her threat. She informed me she had sent an email before the holiday saying she was not taking the complaint further; I had received nothing from her. The call ended and I felt relief but also sadness. The trust on both sides had been broken and neither of us felt safe enough to see if it could be mended. As trust is a crucial element of the therapeutic relationship, I felt there was no possibility of continuing our work together.

She contacted me again three months later, asking if we could resume therapy. I have two supervisors, one who I take the majority of my clients to, who I feel supported by consistently on a day-to-day basis. I also regularly see another supervisor who I bring my more complex trauma clients to. She has years of experience with the most damaged and troubled clients that are ever going to appear in the therapy room. She also happens to be an expert in client complaints, certainly not from choice, but because this group of clients, who are in extreme need of therapeutic help, are also the most likely to fear power, have the least control in their lives and the most suppressed anger to be triggered. They are, not surprisingly, also the most likely to make unsubstantiated complaints. With the guidance of this supervisor, I did some deep internal questioning and sent an email saying I had given the prospect of us continuing our work together much thought. I acknowledged the repair that had taken place since the events before Christmas. I also owned my inability to overcome completely my feelings regarding her threats and therefore did not feel I could be her therapist in the future. I explained that the trust on both sides had been damaged and I could not work to the best of my ability if I was fearful. I stressed this was my failing, it was in no way intended to punish, it was the only way I could find to be truthful and professionally ethical. I offered help with finding a new therapist and sent my best wishes for her future.

Her reply was immediate, conciliatory and accepting. I think she heard the truth in my language, I was being authentic and speaking human to human with her. I owned my inability to continue working with her and showed my concern for her future. It is possible this was a form of repair for the rupture, but there was so much more work that could have been done.

I do not think this had to be the final outcome. There was no actual basis for the formal complaint and the hurt caused could have been contained within the therapeutic relationship. If I had trusted my governing body to make a quick assessment and intention of support, I would have been happy to fold this rupture back into the work and possibly my client would have found it immensely helpful. What I feared was an investigation that would interrupt my practice for months, causing ongoing distress to me and my other clients and possible long-term damage to my reputation and self-belief. As a self-employed therapist in private practice, the ultimate conclusion could also end in complete loss of earnings.

It has always seemed dangerous to me that the entire psychotherapeutic profession, from counsellors to psychoanalysts, is completely unregulated by the government. Currently, anyone can practise as a psychotherapist. After years of lobbying by collective professional bodies, on the 6 March 2020 in a House of Lords debate it was stated, 'The Government currently has no plans to introduce the statutory regulation of counsellors and psychotherapists.'

The knowledge of how to find a therapist who is fully trained, and a member of a reputable professional body, is not commonly known. I very rarely have clients coming to me because they are aware of my qualifications or which professional bodies I am a member of; they often say they liked what I said on my website or they just liked my photograph. A few years ago, I started working with a client who had been severely retraumatized by her last 'therapist'. She had been reluctant to trust again, but because of a desperate need to ease the pain she was in, she decided to take a risk. I was shocked when she described what had happened with her previous therapist and asked her if she would mind me knowing his name. I could find no listing for this person on any training school or professional body. It is likely that he was/is practising with absolutely no training. The worrying thing is, because there is no independent organization to complain to and this person is not a member of any professional body, there is no way of making a complaint about the people most likely to do damage to innocent clients. The damage an untrained person could do to a client, without any redress, is potentially devastating.

I am in no way saying that fully qualified therapists are above mistakes or wrongdoings. We are in a profession that historically has many examples of arrogant therapists 'experimenting' on clients and doing serious harm. The very nature of this relationship between client and therapist can lead to strong emotional confusions. Without a therapist doing enough ongoing personal therapy or having a skilful supervisor whom they are able to be honest with, horrendous mistakes can happen.

Currently counselling and psychotherapy training varies widely in length, areas of study and rigour. The main professional accrediting bodies also vary hugely in requirements and ongoing vigilance. Deliberate and unconscious mistakes need to be investigated if we are to protect some of the most vulnerable members of our society. A robust complaints procedure is vitally important. It is my belief, if there was a government regulating body to investigate complaints about any counsellor or psychotherapist, our individual professional bodies could defend their members better and the clients would have an independent committee looking into their complaints. It would also bring all training and professional organizations up to the same standards. It seems unlikely that one organization can fully represent the client and the therapist.

Another interesting angle of this debate is 'who does the therapist complain to about the client?' I worked with a client who, on her last session, presented me with a hardback book she had written, documenting her therapeutic journey. It was self-published, the hardback cover decorated with one of her drawings done whilst in therapy. She informed me that she had only printed two copies, one for me and one for her, but was thinking of publishing it if I agreed. I always suggest to clients they keep a therapy journal. I inform them that it is a useful tool for processing the physical and emotional reactions in the sessions and a place to put down thoughts and feelings that surface between them. Some clients will bring this to each session and read bits from it, others I never hear what they have written, but will share how important they find it to have something to look back on. This book was different, it read like transcripts of each session. As she hadn't recorded them, much of the dialogue was her interpretation of what we said, rather than our actual words. It was overly complimentary and implied she had been completely healed in eight months. This was someone with a complex history of trauma and abuse. She had been in care most of her young life and had been an inpatient on psychiatric wards after serious suicide attempts. Our ending was because of her financial situation and not, in my understanding, because she had come to the end of the work we were doing.

I took this book home and read it, so she already had my undivided attention for longer than her last session. I spent time considering how I felt about this and how worried I was for her. I made process notes about the transference and countertransference in the presenting of the book. I spoke to my supervisor and made a decision to thank her for the book but stated that I would not give my permission for it to be published. I heard nothing for a month and then I had a more assertive email saying she was going to publish anyway, but I could help edit it with her if I chose. I interpreted this as her unconscious desire to continue working with me but also a grandiose need, from her shamed and damaged self, to avoid feelings of powerlessness. Her need of me was possibly unbearable and she was trying to find a less shaming way for contact. 'What leads to chronic shame is unrepaired disconnection between parent and child' the child is 'likely to conclude, consciously or unconsciously, "There is something wrong with what I need – with my needy self" (DeYoung 2015, p. 20).'

She had made it very clear she could no longer afford therapy so I did not feel I could invite her to return without possibly creating more shame. I also did not want a blow by blow account of our sessions being published when I felt it was such a misrepresentation of my work. I contacted a lawyer, who said I had a strong case to stop the publication but I was halted by my professional responsibility to do no harm. The aggressive act of suing a former client felt as if it would undermine all the work we had done together. I also knew how fragile this person was and feared for her safety. In the end, I contacted another therapist I knew, who worked at a mental health and well-being centre where I knew this client attended a regular group. I did not give any details, I just said I had come to an ending with this person and I was concerned for her. I asked if she could look out for her at the next group meeting and possibly offer a one to one support session. I then came to the conclusion that I had to walk away from the whole thing. I have no idea if the book is published or if it is negatively impacting on my career. I am satisfied with my decision but, throughout this time, I did not feel there was help for me professionally from anywhere.

I am passionate about the work I do, I thank my amazing training every day and the many specific trainings I have attended since. I am supported by theory, experience and two excellent supervisors. Having said that, I often rely on a gut feeling when responding to a client. I do not want my first thought to be one of 'playing safe', but to be free to channel all my skills and expertise for the benefit of that client. I believe totally in the clients' right to complain if they are unhappy with the treatment they receive. I would hope, in the first instance, I had created a space in which they could bring that into the room. When that is not an option there has to be a system that supports both therapist and client to work through the problem. In cases of possible gross misconduct, each person involved deserves respectful enquiry and appropriate response. I do not think we have a system in this country that supports this properly. All too often the person who suffers the most is the client who complains. I believe that the fear of a formal complaint is frequently restricting the creativity of therapists, and supervisors are preoccupied with avoiding possible investigations. This fear can stop us being authentic and from channelling our training and experience into interventions in the consulting room which enable the client to understand and address their deepest issues. The cement of successful relationships is the ability to work through conflict. If the client does not get the chance to do this, either because the therapist is avoiding it or does not want to work with clients who complain, it results in a failing of the very people who need us the most.

CHAPTER 3

Love and hate in the time of Covid: who will watch the watchmen?

Anne Kearns

This chapter looks at what it means to be a member of a professional community and explores the power relationship between the clinician and the professional body and that between the clinician and the client in the context of a recent complaint.

The author's doctoral research highlighted concerns that in their desire to protect the public, professional organizations seem to have lost sight of the need to support – and in some cases protect – their members, particularly against complainants who may use formal complaints procedures to achieve unconscious aims such as to seek revenge on or restitution from a figure from their past.

This research (Kearns, 2006, 2007/2011) also raised the concern that the procedures governing ethical complaints against psychotherapists and counsellors in the UK did not adequately address the complexities of the therapeutic relationship, including the reality that psychotherapists and counsellors often work with people whose ability to relate has been significantly impaired. The author's recent experience indicates that the current system may do more to fuel the complainant's distress than to contain it. The chapter proposes a way forward that may help to diffuse situations arising from potentially explosive complaints in order to support both the practitioner and the client.

Introduction

At the beginning of March 2020, just as the reality of Covid-19 was beginning to dawn on Western Europe, a client made a phone call to my accrediting body to inquire about my membership status. The phone call, though, was not made to the Membership team; it was made to Complaints. A conversation with a case manager led the client to infer that I had to be prevented from practising and that the client needed to take on this task in order to protect others and that is what he attempted to do.

Background to the story

The impetus for this chapter came from various stalking phenomena experienced by me and certain supervisees which began during the Covid-19 lockdowns where research has shown there was an increase in stalking behaviours facilitated by technology (Bracewell, Hargreaves & Stanley, 2020) The 'client' and 'his behaviours' described here are composites of these shared experiences. There is no 'Ian'. But I have used 'him' to highlight flaws in the management of complaints made by dysregulated clients as well as issues faced by British therapists working in the EU.

After many years of practice in the UK, I largely retired and moved to France, while continuing to supervise and to work as an expert witness. As it became locally known that I was a retired psychotherapist, I was also occasionally approached to do some short-term counselling work and to help couples with the problems associated with living in a foreign country.

Talking my new situation through with the membership department of my accrediting body, I decided to register as a 'Non-Clinical Member. This allowed me to keep abreast of developments in the field, to ascribe to a code of ethics, to have a link with a professional organization and retain my UK professional insurance, while no longer maintaining a regular clinical practice.[1]

However, with the approach of Brexit, in 2018 I was informed by my UK insurers that underwriters were not willing to continue to cover British therapists working in the EU. I therefore registered with the French civil authorities as offering psychological counselling ('psychotherapist' being a protected title in France), which meant that any complaint relating to my work with individuals or couples would be subject to French civil law (This situation, or a version of it, will apply to an increasing number of practitioners working in the EU). I got my practice insured and thought nothing further of it. After further discussion with the Accrediting Body about my professional activities, I retained my non-clinical membership status.

'Ian'

'Ian' was referred to me by a local GP. He was British, in crisis, and desperate to see an experienced, English-speaking therapist. I explained to Ian that I was no longer registered as a psychotherapist in the UK but that I remained a non-clinical member and was registered as a psychological counsellor in France. Ian was happy to work with me on this basis.

We had worked together for over a year – sometimes on Zoom – when following a concert tour, Ian had to self isolate for 14 days. Instead of continuing to meet on Zoom he wrote to terminate treatment, thanking me for my hard work and offering to meet for a beer some-day. Before I had a chance to respond I received another email from Ian outlining various concerns. He also asked who I was registered with. I replied that I took his concerns seriously and would discuss them with a colleague, and offered the opportunity to discuss his concerns in the presence of a third party. Ian declined. I also reiterated that I was a non-clinical member of a UK accrediting body, which he already knew.

And so began what turned out to be over a year of my receiving – but not responding to –an onslaught of emails, often containing sexually explicit content and ranging from declarations of love to expressions of his belief that he had been given a mandate by my UK accrediting body to stop me from practising and harming anyone else.[5]

The accrediting body

After receiving an email from Ian telling me that he was informed by my accrediting body I 'should not be practising' I phoned the accrediting body to ask what exactly had been said. A rather nervous-sounding young woman told me that she would have contacted me to see if I was misrepresenting my practise but that, having spoken to me, she was satisfied that I was not.

The following day, the GP who referred Ian to me phoned to say a disturbing email had come from Ian showing him a draft complaint that my accrediting body, allegedly, asked him to submit. The GP said he was just letting me know this as a courtesy and would not respond as he didn't understand why he had been sent this. I phoned my insurers to let them know that the accrediting body had apparently agreed to accept a complaint about my practise, even though, since I was not on their register, my insurers said the accrediting body had no jurisdiction over it. The insurers asked me to confirm this with the accrediting body. For the following six weeks, that was what I attempted to do.

Communication was slowed down by staff having to work at home due to the lockdown. This, however, could not explain why the complaints staff refused to answer whether or not they had asked Ian to submit a complaint. I made regular attempts in writing to get an answer to my question. I tried every possible way of persuading them to help me to help Ian, who I believed was in a dissociative state. I also put to them that I was being bombarded by un-wanted communications from Ian and that it was beginning to make me ill.

My last written request was made after I received an email from Ian asking for a closing session, I replied that before I could agree to this I would need to consult with my insurers and the Accrediting Body. Even though the colleagues with whom I consulted were unanimous in their advice not to agree to such a meeting, I was considering the possibility of doing so to see if I could help Ian. My insurers were adamant that I could not do this if Ian was being encouraged by the Accrediting Body to make a formal complaint. My final email to the complaints department explaining that I couldn't agree to meet with Ian unless I knew about the status of any potential complaint against me went unanswered.

'Professional' organizations?

In the UK, the title of 'psychotherapist' is generic and is not protected, unlike psychologist or psychiatrist. As a supervisor of 'psychotherapists', I consult and advise on the work of psychiatrists, whose psycho-therapy practice is monitored by the General Medical Council (GMC), psychotherapists registered with the United Kingdom Council for Psychotherapy (UKCP), psychotherapists who are members of the British Association for Counselling and Psychotherapy (BACP) and psychotherapists who have emerged from the human potential movement of the 1970s who do not belong to any body at all. I also supervise counselling and clinical psychologists who call themselves psychotherapists who are members of the British Psychological Society (BPS), whose practice is now monitored by the Health Care Professions Council (HCPC).

In 2013, the BACP's voluntary register was accredited by the Professional Standards Authority for Health and Social Care (PSA). This was the first register of its kind to be accredited under a scheme set up by the Department of Health, administered by an independent body and accountable to Parliament. The UKCP's National Register of Psychotherapists has existed since the early 1990s and, although the competition between these two voluntary registers is mainly political and finance-driven, psychotherapists registered with the UKCP have undergone training at Masters level whereas the requirements for BACP registration are not as strict. Furthermore, the BACP makes no distinction between the term 'counsellor' and 'psychotherapist', whereas the UKCP sees counsellors as having had a less rigorous training than psychotherapists who are viewed as having an ability to work in more depth.

The BACP website says that the organization exists for 'one simple reason – counselling changes lives'.[2] They call themselves the professional association for members of the counselling professions in the UK. One must assume that because the 'P' in their acronym stands for psychotherapy, they see psychotherapists as members of the counselling professions. Do not be lulled by their rather airbrushed reason to exist. In a 2016 case that appeared before Mr Justice Mostyn for judicial review, where the BACP had sought to adjudicate a complaint that had already been adjudicated by the UKCP, the judge launched a scathing attack on the BACP for the 'dogged and obstinate' manner in which it pursued the claimant and criticized it for being 'impervious to pleas to act reasonably and fairly'. In his summary he compared their complaints procedure to that of the Star Chamber.[3]

The UKCP's website claims that they 'are the leading organization for the education, training, accreditation and regulation of psychotherapists and psychotherapeutic counsellors in the UK.'[4] This is slightly misleading as the education and training of psychotherapists is done at institutes and universities whose trainings are accredited by the various colleges of the UKCP. The BACP also accredits trainings but you can become a member of the BACP without having graduated from a BACP accredited course. In fact you can sit an online exam for the Certificate of Proficiency (CoP) which claims to be 'a standardized assessment of the skills, knowledge and abilities required to be a professional counsellor or psychotherapist' representing the 'minimum level of competence that clients have a right to expect.'[5] The CoP may be taken up to three times. Failure at the third attempt will result in the candidate's membership being cancelled. After six months one can apply to rejoin but must first sit and pass the CoP.

I think it's safe to conclude that to talk about the 'profession' of psychotherapy is to enter into the realm of tautology and myth. There *is* no profession of psychotherapy. Psychotherapy is what we *do*. Having said that there is not much consensus about *how* we should do it. Collectively we have a way to go before we can reach consensus as to who we *are* and how we agree to be regulated.

The panopticon

One reason for having a formalized profession is to support practices and principles that are specific to that profession, as well as to maintain a body of knowledge and expertise that sets the profession apart from other activities in a way that is recognizable to the public. Professional membership is more than a tacit agreement about what constitutes professional practice, but an assurance that those practices serve to achieve a societal good and are enshrined in an ethical code of conduct. This creates at least two relationships. The first is an intimate, therapeutic relationship, which research shows to be more about how the therapist *is* as opposed to what the therapist knows or does.[6] Despite attempts to engage the client as an equal participant, the therapist may be perceived to hold the power. The second relationship is with other professionals who sign up to a 'body' that is assigned the power in the area of ethical and training standards and monitors what a professional knows and does.

Professional practices have what is called ontological intelligibility. In other words they usually arise from a perceived *reason* to be (someone's good idea) and then evolve to be considered a *necessity* to be. It's a bit like the story of why someone cuts the end of the roast before putting it in the pan. When asked why they do this their answer is because their mother always did it that way. But if you ask granny she will tell you that she did it that way because she did not have a big enough pan.

By professional practices I refer not only to clinical practices, about which there is wide disagreement in the psychotherapy world[7] but also to the 'practical' approach taken by the organizations who regulate psychotherapists.

Jeremy Bentham (1748-1832), the utilitarian philosopher, proposed that a perfect system of observation (Bentham, 1995) would allow one guard in an institution to see the whole situation at any given time. Since this is not possible in all systems – let's take professional practice as an example – there is a need for what Bentham called 'relays' of observers in which 'data' is passed from the lower to the higher level. In a prison, the guards cannot always see each inmate, but from the panopticon – a tower where one guard can choose which part of the situation to view at any given moment – inmates never know if they are being watched so they need always to behave as if they are being observed. Control, then, is achieved by the possibility of being seen rather than being constantly supervised or restrained. But, as the Roman poet Juvenal in the 2nd century asked in a satirical poem which told the story of guards being seduced by one of their captives, 'Who will watch the watchmen?' (*Quis custodiet ipsos custodes?*)

The UK has two main organizations that 'govern' and 'monitor' the practice of their psychotherapist members. Membership, however, is not compulsory. Practitioners who become members of at least one of these organizations accept their power to regulate their practice and to adjudicate complaints. They become the panopticon. As members, we agree to being watched, monitored and governed.

Most practitioners, though, do not become interested in the complaints procedures of their professional organizations until they have a complaint made against them; by which time it is too late to question those procedures.

I believe complaint procedures are often not fit for purpose, and that they need serious and urgent alteration in order to be suitable for supporting the unique relationship between therapist and client/patient, which we call therapeutic relationships. This is particularly true for clients whose ability to relate has been significantly impaired, by often hideous childhood trauma.

Who will watch the watchmen?

The Health and Social Care Act (2012) gave the Professional Standards Authority (PSA) the responsibility for setting standards to accredit voluntary registers as well as to apply conditions and suspend or remove an accrediting bod's accreditation.

In 2018 the BACP's accreditation by the PSA was delayed due to issues that were raised in the 2016 judicial review by the High Court. The panel's concerns were largely about the number of complaints that were initially rejected but then resubmitted following advice from case managers as well as the support offered to complainants going through the complaints process.

The UKCP's accreditation with the PSA was suspended in November 2015 due to concerns that the UKCP fell short of being committed to protecting the public and in inspiring public confidence. The UKCP did not notify its members of this suspension until the day before the deadline for responding to the PSA's concerns about their Complaints and Conduct Process Rules (CCPR). These concerns were addressed and the UKCP was reinstated but the process of hastily-thought-through procedures and a lack of transparency should be of interest to its current members in light of its stance on exploring alternative routes to complaint resolution.

In the PSA's 2019 Annual Review of the UKCP's complaints procedures it was noted that the previous year's review had expressed concern that the UKCP advertised a formal 'Alternative Dispute Resolution' (ADR) but that these procedures were unclear and seemed also to be unavailable. The PSA issued a recommendation to the UKCP that its ADR be made accessible to the public, or otherwise removed from its website. The UKCP confirmed it had amended its website to remove references to the ADR procedure. When asked to confirm its plans for ADR the UKCP replied:

'We do not have plans to develop a formal ADR policy – we do explain to registrants (for complaints that do not indicate unsuitability to be on the UKCP register) that they should talk to their therapist in the first instance (to save the therapeutic relationship).'[8]

Are we to understand that when asked to make its ADR policy *more* accessible the UKCP's response was to discontinue it and explain to registrants [*sic*] – I assume they mean complainants – that they should talk to their therapists in order to 'save the therapeutic relationship'. This wording seems to imply that the client has some responsibility to 'save' the therapeutic relationship. I suggest that the administrators who are on the front line of fielding complaints from the public have a shared responsibility to support the therapy to continue where at all possible.[9]

The UKCP's claim to explain to potential complainants the benefits of talking to the therapist is a bit misleading. Its website's advice on how to make a complaint does say that the simplest way of resolving disagreements or concerns is to speak to your therapist to 'see if they can put things right'. They recommend that 'you try to resolve your concerns with your therapist before lodging a formal complaint'. They suggest to potential complainants who may not 'feel comfortable' talking to their therapist about their concerns the option of using UKCP's formal Complaints and Conduct Process. Potential complainants are invited to discuss by telephone the 'most suitable options for [their] concerns' with a member of the Complaints and Conduct Team. And herein I believe lies a problem that may unwittingly escalate ruptures rather than resolve them.

Speaking frankly?

The French philosopher Foucault (2011) was interested in *parrhesia* or the courageous act of truth telling, not to advocate for free speech but rather to explore the moral and political position one must occupy in order to take the risk to speak truthfully.

From his emails to me and those to colleagues where I was copied in, it is abundantly clear that Ian believed – and may still believe – that he had a duty to tell the truth and to protect others. Some 10 weeks after his first contact with the complaints case manager Ian sent me an email where he revealed that not only did he feel abused by me but he also felt betrayed by the accrediting body and let it be known that the press would be contacted to expose their failings. Ian was grateful that his new therapist was helping him see how abusive I had been and had started a blog to find others who had felt abused by their therapists. Additionally, he wrote that when he had contacted the accrediting body the person on the phone agreed that I had abused my power. Ian also came to believe that the accrediting body had written to me to tell me to stop practising with clients. One of the websites where my details are listed contacted me as ask if this was true so I can only assume that they were contacted by Ian.

I do not know what was said by 'the person on the phone' but I cannot imagine that they had agreed I had abused my power. The accrediting body did not send me a letter telling me to stop practising. In one of the emails I received from a member of the Complaints team, it was suggested to me that I was on the wrong membership category and that I should discuss this with Membership. As I had discussed this with Membership on two occasions two years apart, I could not see the need to do this again. I wrote to Membership to cancel my non-clinical membership and they wrote back that they were sorry to see me go. It would seem that the watchmen do not always talk to each other.

The way forward

For the last 25 years or so I have been concerned that complaints against psychotherapists and other practitioners of the talking therapies are largely mismanaged from the outset and that this mismanagement is damaging to both the complainants and practitioners. I want to use what was a distressing experience for both me and Ian to find a way forward.

The relationship between client and psychotherapist is in many ways like other relationships except for the boundaries that govern time, payment, dual relationships, indiscriminate self-disclosure and sexual contact. All relationships are subject to chance and change. My demeanour on any given day can be influenced by any number of non-clinical elements and a client who is particularly sensitive may indeed intuit things about me that I do not choose to express or to share. This sensitivity to the unexpressed effect of the therapist, and to changes to, or intrusions into the therapeutic frame, is particularly relevant when the client has (as was the case with Ian) a history of abuse or a clinical presentation of Complex PTSD (post-traumatic stress disorder) or DID.

Issues such as feeling rejected by changing an appointment time or even gestures of genuine kindness can lead to clinical ruptures. My concern is that these ruptures occur in a context and when they become viewed as 'mistakes' they become freeze-framed. It is my firm belief that clinical ruptures and even some serious errors of judgement can and should be worked through with a skilled third party rather than seen as misdemeanours to be adjudicated and possibly sanctioned.

For people with histories of abuse, the relational conditions of the therapy itself are likely to trigger off earlier relational states that cause the client to re-enact an earlier trauma by complaining about the therapist. The difficulty in helping traumatized people is that they are likely to attribute to the therapist many of the same motives as the perpetrator(s) and to suspect the therapist of exploitative intentions. Herman (1992, pp. 137–8) says that when

> 'the therapist fails to live up to the client's idealized expectations – *as he inevitably will fail* – the patient is often overcome with fury. Because the patient feels as though her life depends upon her rescuer (the therapist) she can not afford to be tolerant; there is no room for human error … there *have to be consequences.*'

With this in mind it should be incumbent upon us to insist that our regulators do not abuse our more vulnerable clients even further. We need procedures that contain the trauma, not exacerbate it. I use my recent experience as an example of how this can happen. People like Ian deserve to have their concerns treated with more understanding of their fragility. For regulators this requires anticipation of that fragility. I do not hold the accrediting body responsible for Ian's behaviour. But it does appear that the case manager answered a question put to her over the telephone without considering the context in which it was being asked and without knowing, for example, the facts of where I lived and worked. Context is key.

The case manager who took Ian's phone call was probably sympathetic and kind. The problem is that remarks that aim to soothe, like 'that sounds as though it was difficult for you' can be interpreted by fragile complainants as acceptance of *their* truth. People who have been abused as children by people in charge have a deep desire to be heard and believed. I would like to see a change in current procedures so that no phone contact is made with potential complainants until they first put their concerns in writing. At that point an assessment could be made by another psychotherapist, not a lay case manager, of the context of the complaint and the possible mental state of the complainant. The complainant could then be encouraged and supported to seek resolution directly with their therapist or the regulator could facilitate conciliation where resolution is not possible.

The handling of a complaint is a complex process that requires attention to complex psychological issues, particularly transference dynamics and cultural issues involving power, race, gender, sexuality and the ability to assimilate information. Addressing these with equanimity in the screening process does not negate the possibility that the complainant may be found to have a genuine grievance.

Telephone contact between complainants and the regulator should no longer be an option, even when 'just' answering apparently straightforward questions or giving information. Practitioners skilled in crisis intervention could take on this role if a member of the public in distress needs help in formulating a complaint or in finding a way forward. We could even create a role for an ombudsman. Any solution must include reinstating and developing procedures for alternative dispute resolution. Many practitioners have the needed skills to make this feasible and could urge their accrediting bodies to make this happen.

Throughout Ian's communications to me and to my various colleagues ran the thread that the new therapist was encouraging his stand against the abuse that he allegedly endured in therapy with me. It is very easy to become confluent with a client's version of what happened in their previous therapy. Indeed, I think it would be useful to research the role of the replacement therapist in supporting a client to complain. I would urge a change to our codes of ethics to require a therapist to communicate with the previous therapist before agreeing to work with a client where no onward referral has been made. I have found that without this contact, the therapist who takes over from a therapist who has 'failed' is likely to be susceptible to a rescue fantasy (Freud, 1957), seeing oneself as the one who will save the client where all others have failed. This can lead to therapeutic omnipotence and the demonizing of the 'guilty party' (Berman, 1993). If we are to be professionals and collegial we owe each other the benefit of the doubt.

Furthermore Anglo-European therapists working in the EU who may be registered with a UK accrediting organization need a more helpful and informative response to clients who may feel the need to check their legitimacy or to complain about their work when that work takes place in a split Europe.

Notes

1. It may interest you to know that one definition of 'active' clinical practice is 'an average of 20 hours per week or 640 hours'.
2. www.bacp.co.uk
3. https://www.kingsleynapley.co.uk/insights/blogs/regulatory-blog/dogged-and-obstinate-bacp-prevented-from-proceeding-to-adjudicate-on-a-complaint-already-disposed-of-by-the-ukcp
4. www.psychotherapy.org.uk/about-ukcp
5. www.bacp.co.uk/membership/registered-membership/certificate-of-proficiency
6. Research on psychotherapy's effectiveness has revealed that the relational qualities of the therapist are more influential on the outcome than any single therapeutic approach (Lambert, 1986; Lambert and Barley, 2001; Heinonen and Nissen-Lie, 2019).
7. When providing theoretical support for a psychotherapist's practical choices when I acted as expert in a Professional Conduct Hearing I drew upon several works published by members of the Institute of Psychoanalysis in Chicago. These were dismissed by one of the panelists – a psychoanalytic psychotherapist – as 'American theories'.
8. www.professionalstandards.org.uk/docs/default-source/accredited-registers/panel-decisions/ukcp-annual-review-2020.pdf?sfvrsn=7a7b7420_6. The Professional Standard's Agency's 2019 Annual Review of the UKCP's complaints procedures is no longer available online; it has been superseded by a document of the same name but dated January 2021. The document quoted was dated November 2019 and is only available on request.
9. Annual review of accreditation 2019/20, UK Council for Psychotherapy (UKCP) November 2019

CHAPTER 4

A constructive way of dealing with conflict

Kay Beaumont

Being investigated following a complaint can be a devastating experience. The process is often adversarial leaving the person being investigated struggling to demonstrate innocence rather than the complainant (or investigators) having to prove their case. It encourages defensiveness and closes down learning. Some years ago a family complained that I had planted false memories of sexual abuse in their daughter. I describe the complaint, its effect on me, on the service user, and my thoughts on how it could have been dealt with more constructively. Clinicians are not above being investigated, but I argue that a persecutory system damages those involved. A restorative justice process, enabling those harmed and those responsible to play a part in understanding what happened, is a constructive way of dealing with conflict.

Introduction

Working with people in a role offering advice, help or therapy is a privilege and can be profoundly rewarding. Satisfaction comes from building trusting relationships, reducing distress so that the person seeking help feels mentally stronger and in control of his/her life. But sometimes relationships break down, service users are dissatisfied and complaints are made. This can be devastating, particularly as a complaints process is frequently adversarial, bureaucratic and at odds with a culture of empathy and compassion. If justice and improved services are the desired outcome, then many of the current systems are seriously lacking.

In the complaint investigation I experienced, no lessons were learned and I was left devastated by the experience. This, and my experience of investigating complaints, has caused me to reflect on how it could be improved. In this paper I will consider what usually takes place when a patient or service user makes a complaint, the complaint made against me, and how a restorative justice model can improve the experience by creating honesty and openness without the absence of responsibility.

Making a complaint

There are three main parties involved in a complaint made by a service user – the agency conducting the complaint, the complainant and the person who is the subject of the complaint. However, there is no equity of power between the three parties. The agency is the most powerful player and its primary concern is to protect its reputation, demonstrate that the complaint process has been followed, and show that it has taken the matter seriously. In many situations, the agency will seek to apportion blame, but this is rarely directed at the agency itself. It is usually directed at the subject of the complaint.

Even where blame is not directed at the subject of the complaint, the experience feels persecutory. The person's reputation is under threat, particularly if s/he is suspended while the investigation takes place. An open and honest discussion becomes impossible in an atmosphere where the subject of the complaint has to prove their innocence. The process encourages an atmosphere of defensiveness rather than one of learning. This adversarial approach does not instil confidence among staff.

If a complaint resolution is to mean anything, the outcome should increase our understanding. In many of the high profile enquiries, the stated desire is to learn the lessons, but blame is more prominent than understanding. My experience is that the recommendations inevitably increase the number of forms to complete, and staff, who are already anxious following the incident, become adept at form filling but lack confidence in decision making. Improving staff confidence by focusing on good practice and paying less attention to bureaucracy and managerialism would be far more beneficial to staff and service users.

Munro and Turnell describe managerialism as an organizational and administrative system where priority is on the economic and management concerns of the employer rather than the needs of service users or staff: 'In many jurisdictions, managerialism has so constrained individual discretion and choice of action that rights-based practice is hard to achieve' (Munro and Turnell, 2018, p. 89).

There will be rare occasions when a staff member intentionally harms someone. This cannot be ignored and the staff member should be referred to the relevant organizations, but the majority of staff want to provide the best care possible and should be listened to when something does not go as expected. An open, resilient employer who listens to staff will create a confident workforce.

The person who initiated the complaint process wants a resolution. There may be hurt and anger behind the complaint, but so often the complainant will want their story to be heard, their experience acknowledged and changes made to the service so that the incident is not repeated. Sadly, so many procedures take a long time and complainants are left not knowing what is happening. This reinforces feelings of hurt and anger and positions become polarized. Added to this, the complainant notices the staff behaving in a defensive manner, and this gets in the way of hearing a true account of what really happened. Sharing stories – the complained about and the complainant – in a safe setting early in the investigation is a starting point for resolving the conflict.

Most complainants are genuine in their pursuit of a resolution, but there are people who make allegations that are simply not true. In these circumstances the agency should support their staff and be honest with the complainant. The complaint against me took place some years ago when I worked as a senior social worker. It highlighted the desire of my employer to protect itself. The pressures on the mental state of a young woman were less important than the influence of an angry family.

Jasmine[1]

Jasmine was a young woman in her twenties, who came to my notice when I and another social worker ran a group for women survivors of sexual abuse. Jasmine had initially disclosed her abuse to staff at a health clinic and was referred for a psychiatric assessment. Following treatment for depression the psychiatrist referred her to our group. Jasmine was intelligent, articulate, and able to express herself verbally and through poems and art. She described appalling abuse from a close family friend throughout her childhood. Her family were regular attenders at a local church and the family friend, Gerald, was the church warden. When she grew up and left home, her relationship with her family became strained. She feared that if she saw her parents this would be a way back into contact with Gerald.

Jasmine kept telephone contact with her parents, who lived a considerable distance away. The telephone contact, she explained, was to prevent them from coming to visit her. Her reasoning was that if they did not hear from her they would be more likely to visit, but there was always an underlying fear that her family and possibly Gerald would visit anyway and so she decided to seek legal advice. She made an independent decision to go to a solicitor, possibly having gained confidence from members of the group. The solicitor wrote to Jasmine's parents and Gerald saying Jasmine wanted no contact.

With advice from members of the community psychiatric team, I continued to see Jasmine when the group finished. Early on it became apparent that honesty and reliability were important to her which helped us build a trusting relationship. It was not my role to investigate or challenge what she was describing. My role was to provide a safe space, listen, help her understand her feelings and promote recovery. Jasmine chose to talk about her abuse without prompting. She still had intrusive thoughts and painful memories, but with support her depression was under control and she was able to work.

Sometime after the solicitor's letter, Jasmine saw Gerald in the distance near the flat she shared with two other young women. She was frightened and contacted the solicitor who wrote again saying she wanted no further contact with him or her parents.

Shortly after the letters were sent, Jasmine said Gerald visited when her flatmates were out, forced his way in and raped her. She did not tell us until a week later when she had become withdrawn, terrified and suicidal. The psychiatric team wanted her admitted to hospital but for complex reasons she had to be admitted to a different hospital with a new psychiatric team. This team were informed that Jasmine wanted no contact with her family or Gerald.

While in hospital, Jasmine's mental state became more stable and she decided to report the rape to the police, but the police were critical of the delay in reporting and lack of forensic evidence because she had destroyed the clothes she had worn at the time. The police also embarked on a strange mission to investigate her, and told me that a woman with mental health issues was an unreliable witness. At this point Jasmine withdrew from the investigation, finding it too intrusive and felt the police did not believe her. Instead she spoke to her solicitor who wrote again to Gerald and her parents, copied to the hospital psychiatric team, stating Jasmine wanted no contact.

Jasmine's parents ignored the letter, found out her whereabouts from her flatmates and met with her psychiatrist. I understand he gave them my name. On hearing from nurses that her parents had been to the hospital and spoken to her psychiatrist, Jasmine immediately discharged herself and went to stay in a women's refuge. This hospital team had no further involvement in her care.

The complaint

Shortly after Jasmine discharged herself I received a copy of a complaint letter from Jasmine's parents sent to my employer (a local authority) and also copied to various professional, social care, health and political organizations and the False Memory Society. The letter stated that I had breached professional boundaries, grossly abused my authority, prevented their daughter from having contact with them and through regression therapy had planted false memories of abuse carried out by their close friend Gerald. The letter had an attachment written by Jasmine's flatmates stating that I had visited Jasmine at home at midnight and was having a sexual relationship with her. I found the letter and attachment devastating because it contained so much misinformation, and challenged my professional conduct. Apart from the false accusations directed at me, there were outright lies, for example, her parents said they had enjoyed a lovely day out with their daughter when she was clearly in hospital and had not left the ward.

I assumed my local authority would not accept this as a complaint partly because it contained so many claims that could be easily refuted, but also because it came from a third party, and the service user was an adult who categorically did not want to make a complaint. Additionally, a solicitor taking instructions from her had written three times informing her parents she wanted no contact with them or Gerald. Instead the agency wrote to me fully intending to follow up the complaint:

> the department needs to respond to the suggestion that you breached your professional boundaries and grossly abused your authority. You are aware that the complainants provide some information to support their claim and indicate that they have support from other agencies in this matter.

I can assure you that the time taken in preparing a detailed report is essential to ensure that we are adequately prepared for any action taken by the complainant following receipt of the response.' The last sentence suggested fear of legal action. The idea that therapists were planting false memories received a great deal of media coverage which I believe added to nervousness in the local authority.

I was informed the complaint fell outside the usual remit but the agency decided to proceed because they considered the allegations to be so serious. Early in the investigation, Jasmine wrote independently giving a detailed account of her abuse which she said continued until she was 18 years old. The abuse, she explained, had never been forgotten, and I was not the first person she told. This had no effect on the way the process was to be conducted.

There is no doubt in my mind that the agency felt intimidated by the publicity surrounding false memories, an alleged abuser who was a respected member of the church, and parents, who presented as successful professionals. Many agencies were mentioned in the letter from the parents, but in the end none were prepared to support them other than possibly the False Memory Society. The complaint was eventually concluded after five months. I was the second from last person to be interviewed. This was after the parents, flatmates, managers and colleagues. Jasmine was the last. It was alarming to find out that in planning her interview the investigators had not recognized Jasmine's vulnerability. There was no understanding of the stress she was experiencing and no specific ideas about how to support her. In the end, I found someone to be her advocate and supporter at the interview, someone she already knew which she said was helpful.

I was told the delay was because the flatmates did not want to be interviewed and cancelled appointments, although one of them did reluctantly agree to be interviewed. No evidence was found to support the allegations. I was not offered the opportunity of discussing the outcome, although the parents were invited to discuss the findings, an invitation they did not take up. They had no further contact with the local authority.

The effect of the complaint on Jasmine

Jasmine told us that as a child Gerald said he would destroy any person she told about the abuse, and she believed this was happening to me, which meant we had a strange responsibility towards each other. I wanted her to survive this attack, because attack is what it felt like, and I needed her to see that I could survive too, but we watched as she became depressed and suicidal.

The situation reached a crisis when Jasmine attended an outpatient appointment with her psychiatrist. He was extremely concerned and contacted me. At the time I wrote, *(the psychiatrist) thought Jasmine felt completely hopeless and intended ending her life after her interview date regarding the complaint. She was worried I would lose my job, and said she had things to do and when they were completed there was no reason to stay alive. The psychiatrist found her extremely withdrawn, and asked me to see her.* I discussed her safety with the psychiatrist. As with any seriously depressed patient, we considered hospital admission, but bearing in mind her previous experience, we knew she would not agree, and the prospect of formal detention under the Mental Health Act 1983 was out of the question because she would lose control when the focus of her treatment had been on helping her regain control of her life. Also, if we proceeded along this route, we would have to consult her nearest relative. Legally this would be the elder of her parents. The nearest relative could be removed legally, but this would take time and would draw her family into the process. Another problem was that the ward was a mixed ward with mainly male patients two of whom were very ill and disinhibited, and the psychiatrist was concerned Jasmine would feel unsafe.

The following day Jasmine came to see me. She was very withdrawn and tense. There was no eye contact, her body was turned away from me, and it was difficult to engage her in conversation. I imagined she was hearing the hostile voice of Gerald. On previous occasions she told me that when she was feeling low she would hear his voice and that a gentle voice in the 'real world' had a calming effect reducing the impact of the voice in her head. With this in mind, despite the lack of response, I continued to talk, constantly reassuring her that I would not lose my job, that I was OK and that we wanted her to be safe. My profound feeling was that she did not want to live but was unsure about whether she wanted to die. I had observed this in service users before. In a desperate state they did not want to live but wanted a reason not to die, and that usually came through a connection with a person. With Jasmine I had to reach her and give a reason to live beyond the complaint interview date.

The reason was indeed small. My birthday was two weeks after her complaint interview. In more normal times I would never have brought this into a discussion with a service user, but desperate measures were required, and without any prior planning I said that to celebrate this significant birthday my social work colleague and I thought of having a lunch with the members of the survivor's group Jasmine had attended. I stressed the importance of her being there. There was an initial silence as she absorbed the words. In my notes I wrote *Her face changed. It was as if there was a release of energy and she began to weep.* She said she would be at the group meeting, and as she was very reliable, I knew she would. I reported this back to the psychiatrist and we arranged for members of the community mental health team to phone Jasmine each evening just for a few minutes between 7.00 and 8.00 p.m., the most difficult time of the day for her. They knew to speak to her in a gentle voice to counter the negative voice of Gerald.

Jasmine's interview with the investigators went ahead supported by her advocate and after her initial fear, she told me she was able to say what she wanted, and felt relieved. The group meeting and celebration took place and was surprisingly pleasant. I felt we were over this crisis. Her psychiatrist wrote:

'I am pleased to say that following a very concerning recent period, I found her (Jasmine) to be improved today. She was more talkative and her interaction was better. It was a weight off her shoulders to get through the meeting regarding the allegations about Kay Beaumont made by her parents. She feels that she did not let Kay down, and did not find the meeting particularly stressful.'

He suggested a referral to a psychologist.
The psychologist worked with Jasmine over several weeks, mainly

addressing the issue of Gerald's voice, and wrote:

> She (Jasmine) has been examining the idea that the content of
> the voice is perhaps relevant to what she actually says to herself
> on occasions. Interestingly, she has found this quite a comforting
> idea and finds it easier to dispute the voice believing that it is
> actually her own thoughts rather than Gerald's.

After the complaint, Jasmine's mental state became more stable, and
we were able to acknowledge her courage in standing up to Gerald and
her family.

The effect of the complaint on me

Jasmine and I were not kept informed about the complaint process,
and because my line managers were either investigating me or going to
be interviewed about me, they could not discuss the case. In fact, my
employer left me without any support, although eventually agreed that
I should get help from an external therapist, which was enormously
helpful. I also sought advice from a professional organization, but the
person allocated to assist me seemed overwhelmed by it all and was
frankly unhelpful. I was consumed by the complaint for several months
to an extent where I felt I was suffering from a form of secondary trauma.

The phenomenon of traumatic counter-transference, as experienced
by therapists, social workers and clinicians working with people who
have experienced severe abuse, is recognized (Herman, 1992). I found
listening to Jasmine's accounts of extreme sexual abuse, degradation
and even torture deeply troubling but the complaint introduced other
intense feelings. Like her, I felt helpless and vulnerable. I also felt split
into fragments. Part of me was invested in keeping a distressed young
woman alive and feeling worthy of living, while another was furiously
trying to defend myself. I was also expected to carry on with the daytime
supervision and management of staff as if nothing had happened.

Gerald and Jasmine's family permeated everything, from the voices
in Jasmine's head to the letters of complaint, yet I could not discuss
any aspect of my feelings with my line managers because they were
involved in the investigation. This left me holding the responsibility for
the case on my own. In fact my anger was not directed towards Gerald

or the complainants, and neither was Jasmine's. My feelings of anger were towards my service and managers, while Jasmine described feeling deeply hurt rather than angry that her family chose to support Gerald and not her.

The investigation process and how it could be improved

It could be argued that the complaint should not have proceeded at all as discussed earlier, but I shall consider how a restorative approach could have been used and would have been an improvement.

Restorative justice brings those harmed and those responsible into communication in a fair and unbiased way. The process ensures everyone affected is involved in repairing the harm and finding a positive way forward. It is about a process of investigating conflict, but it is also about the values underpinning any investigation – the values of openness, fairness and respect with an outcome that leads to greater understanding.

In this complaint, it would not have been possible to bring the participants together. Gerald was not a party to the complaint, and would not be included, but Jasmine would not have agreed to meet the complainants, her family. The interviews would therefore have to take place separately, but working in an adapted restorative way, the experience would have been less stressful.

To create a sense of fairness, this investigation should be conducted by two people with no connection to me or the case, but with an understanding of mental health and sexual abuse, people who are open-minded, not driven by the need to look for blame or compelled simply to protect the local authority. Good preparation and communication is vital so that trust can be gained. Jasmine, the service user, is the most vulnerable and her mental health is of paramount concern. To reduce her anxiety, she must be the first person interviewed, followed by me to establish my professional view of what had taken place, and finally the family should be interviewed.

The investigators must write to the participants introducing themselves, explaining the process and ensuring the participants are kept informed throughout. Their neutrality will need to be emphasized, confidentiality explained and each participant invited to bring a supporter to their interview. Beforehand, the participants will be told the sort of questions they will be asked – open questions about what happened, who has been affected, and how they felt. The process would be about investigating the complaint and not whether abuse had or had not taken place. This would need to be emphasized. The interview is an opportunity for each person to be listened to, treated with respect and not judged. This applies to everyone, including the family.

In a usual restorative process, the investigators would identify who has been harmed. This is difficult in this case as the allegations in the complaint are unfounded, but instead the investigators should consider who has been harmed by the complaint. I would argue that harm was caused to both Jasmine and me as a result of the way the local authority managed it. A discussion with the investigators after the process was completed would have been a way of addressing this. Jasmine and her advocate should also have been offered the chance of a post-investigation meeting so that she could explain how it had impacted on her. If this had been adopted, Jasmine may not have felt so overwhelmed that she no longer wanted to live, and I would have felt more valued as a professional, less isolated and more supported.

The family wanted the focus to be on blame and punishment and without this it is difficult to predict how they would have responded. Gerald and Jasmine's family were known and respected in their local community and any suggestion of child sexual abuse was impossible for them to accept. Unlike me, the family were offered the chance of meeting with the investigators, but turned it down.

There are people who will find a restorative process difficult, people, like Jasmine's family, who refused to acknowledge the harm their daughter had experienced and wanted retribution and blame rather than engaging in a conversation. This was a firm and unmovable position. There was no openness of discussion or self-reflection. Despite this, the investigators should listen to and respect their contribution.

After the complaint

The complaint process went against all my principles of working with service users. Jasmine's family had been allowed to intrude into her life despite her views clearly expressed through her solicitor and directly to the investigators. Our emphasis had been on empowering her so she could take control of her life and determine her own future, yet the complaint reduced her to a child still under the power of her family and her alleged abuser. At no point did I or any other member of the team tell her not to communicate with her parents. This was her decision following discussions with her solicitor.

This complaint took place some years ago; I hope some aspects will be different now. However, I still believe people seen to be powerful can exert undue influence. Colleagues and former colleagues I have spoken to say that complaints continue to leave people feeling persecuted and deskilled, but there are enlightened organizations changing this.

Restorative approaches to address complaints

Restorative justice can be delivered in many ways and is shown to be effective in the criminal justice system where victims report high levels of satisfaction (Victim Support, 2010). It has been particularly successful in schools and on Youth Offending Panels, and regarded as an effective way of developing empathy and responsibility among young people. This is in contrast to an adversarial approach which tends to focus on blame and shame, but which rarely brings about positive change because it creates defensiveness and resentment. 'Restorative processes give children and young people the insight and skills to deal creatively and positively with conflict' (Graham Robb, quoted in Cook, 2014).

A restorative approach needs to be part of a wider organization culture based on openness, consistency and valuing staff. An organization that has adopted restorative principles will be resilient, and supportive towards staff so that when problems arise, which they inevitably will, they can be discussed openly. NHS organizations, like Barts Health NHS Trust and Mersey Care who work restoratively, have based their policies on the work of Professor S. Dekker, based in Queensland, Australia (NHS Resolution, 2019). Professor Dekker's approach is systemic and focuses on the systems and organizations involved rather than assigning blame to front line workers and clinicians. At the outset organizations need to decide what they hope to achieve from an investigation. 'If blame is the goal, any investigation tends to stop after the "culprit(s)" have been identified and the opportunity for learning is lost.' (NHS Resolution, *2019*, p. 23).

In my experience, having worked restoratively in schools and as a panel member in a youth offending service, sometimes the most resistant people can find comfort providing there is good preparation beforehand and skilled facilitators. Reconciliation comes from honesty, accepting our own vulnerability, treating others respectfully and acknowledging that it will be difficult.

Conclusion

No overall lessons were learned by the local authority following the complaint against me. There was no organizational understanding. In fact it was never mentioned again so far as I am aware. Both Jasmine and I survived the complaint. In different ways we were abandoned, Jasmine by her family and me by my employer, but we both received support. Jasmine received support from me and the clinical team, and she learned an important lesson, that her alleged abuser and her family could not control everything in her life. I was fortunate to have the support of family and friends and the help of a therapist who worked with survivors of sexual abuse and understood the impact this had on me. But it was also about justice and truth. I was determined that my name should not be tainted by untruths, and that Jasmine had a right to help in a confidential setting without interference from her family.

The experience influenced my practice when I was later employed as a senior manager. Following a serious incident or complaint, I understood that early contact from a senior staff member was important. Gathering staff together to discuss the incident in a supported, non-judgemental setting helped staff talk about what had happened and feel valued. Any serious incident, such as a suicide, is shocking for staff. They are worried about the outcome, in particular thinking whether it could have been prevented and concerned about the inevitable coroner's hearing. But, also a tragedy has occurred and there is a sense of loss because a vulnerable person known to them has died unexpectedly.

Talking to staff and involving them in suggesting improvements rather than top-down management directives is invaluable. Changing from an adversarial response to a restorative way of resolving conflict benefits everyone. It becomes easier to admit when something has gone wrong with an apology and an explanation, and staff will be less fearful. Mersey

Trust reported a 64 per cent reduction in disciplinary cases between 2016 and 2017 as a result of adopting a restorative justice approach to complaints. In summary, 'Having a level of psychological safety, where issues can be raised and addressed before they escalate, is a major factor in improving both patient and staff safety' (NHS Resolution, 2019).

Notes

1. All identifying details of this case have been changed, to protect the anonymity of all the people involved.

CHAPTER 5

Complaints in the field of dissociative disorders: six key categories

Valerie Sinason

It has taken the world time to come to terms with the level of sexual and domestic trauma in peacetime. As late as the 1970s in the UK, child sexual abuse was seen as an extremely rare minority experience by child psychotherapists and others in the National Health Service. Lloyd de Mause (1974) presciently pointed out at that time that the history of childhood was a nightmare which we were only just beginning to emerge from in a few countries. In the 50 years that have followed, our society has slowly had to face the existence of abuse by parents, teachers, social workers, clerics. More recently our society has had to face the existence of organized abuse, the perverse collaboration of parents with others, religious groups and institutions of all kinds. We face the enormity of internet grooming and abuse, the level of attacks on women, abuse of child athletes and actors and adults from all walks of life bravely coming forward over current or retrospective abuse including #MeToo. Every decade we face another aspect of social trauma.

In the last few decades, we have struggled to realize that a minority of abused people develop dissociative disorders, as a defence against trauma. In the three decades I have focused on this work (including founding the Clinic for Dissociative Studies in 1998), I have become aware of a particular range of complaints which characterizes this group. These complaints stem from a recurring narrative, which I would like to explore here.

This narrative happens all over the world. The scenarios below are amalgamations of countless accounts. They are drawn from people I have met, supervised, heard from, complaints I have investigated, and complaints made against me and colleagues over the past three decades, involving the most vulnerable and traumatized people. This is usually about a female patient but occasionally a male. I will use the pronoun 'she' here.

The narrative

A brave woman (although sometimes it is a man) who says she has been sadistically abused since as far back as she can remember, says she is making plans to leave what she calls her abusive home.

Week by week she slowly moves clothes and other items out to the houses of different friends and neighbours who do not know each other. She transports them in different carrier bags and rucksacks so that should one of her hiding places be found, her remaining bits and pieces or plans would be hard to put together. She does all this so that her final exit will not be noted, and she could finally leave with only her usual work bag.

She does this with terror and determination.

She had told her closest friends about the abuse she had suffered within her family, outside of her family and by people her family had hired her out to. And then, on a cold but bright morning, her heart beating louder than her alarm clock, she left the way she always did for work. Her usual breakfast and cup of tea rising inside her, her voice still managed to say, 'See you later' as she closed the front door and walked out at her usual pace on fledgling orphan feet.

Shortly afterwards, having left her home, her job, her town, and before arranging to pick up her clothes and books from all the different safe places they were hidden away in, she attempted the most terrifying part of her plan: she went to the police in her new area. It was not only her own abuse she wished to report but the abuse of other children. There were big names involved, the kind we have all heard, and speaking up was going against everything she'd been brought up to obey.

She did not know then, and many survivors now still do not know, that the police will not investigate crimes from another area: crimes must be reported where they occurred. A stolen car – yes, they can do that – but not rape allegations. Her new local police were concerned for her safety and enabled her to find safe housing. They took video disclosures and statements. But they could not investigate: all the documents and videos were handed over to the police force local to her childhood home, despite the woman's plea that her family were friendly with the local police. Indeed, she alleged senior officers were involved.

Freed from her family whilst the investigation went on, she started treatment. There were several false starts, where professionals, without support or adequate training, were too frightened to work with her; but eventually she found a therapist. She also had the help of a couple of good friends who painstakingly continued to bring her belongings for her, and she was able to further her career hopes.

As time went on, however, she was subject to a few incidents of abuse and intimidation, and there was confusion as to how this happened. After a further serious attack was reported and evidenced more police became involved. Whilst her friends were in hope of a resolution, the police had no hope of a conviction. One officer queried whether the injuries were self-inflicted. Another wondered if she was covering up drunken promiscuity with a rape story. The officers who had previously been involved and felt she was a good witness who deserved to have her case investigated had somehow been moved on, retired or were distinctly uneasy. No one was going to risk their career investigating this case. The woman watched all this with a heartsink: her family were right, they were all above the law and nothing and no one would stop them.

Two more elements were against her: she had Dissociative Identity Disorder (DID[1]) and she was reporting abuse of a ritualistic kind. Both of these made her appear as an unreliable witness. And both posed a problem for police, other professionals and the woman herself, including all her personalities.

A 'personality' who is trauma-bonded to her abusers can write or phone home or give away her new address, not realizing this could lead to other personalities and the shared body being attacked. This in turn could lead to further terror for the main personality and those who knew her. Her friends were dumbfounded and frightened as to how yet another place of asylum had been destroyed. The lack of training in DID and organized and ritualized abuse meant her helpers also ascribed more power to the abusers than was warranted. 'How could her abusers know where she was? They must be so clever,' was the regular assumption and concern from professionals and friends. This led to the secondary traumatization of her professional network, frightened they could be hurt too.

The tragically simple tale of a child conditioned through torture to report her every move and new address was not known at that time. Instead, there was the terrifying narrative of an adult victim with an all-seeing, or even supernatural enemy, who would know wherever and whenever she moved, even if she had a few weeks' clear start when her disappearance really did shock her family.

Nevertheless, her efforts and the support she received were not wasted. While she was still subject to intermittent rapes and assaults, she did, on the whole, live a different kind of life, developing her talents, making some safe relationships and daring to speak about the kind of abuse she had survived. She may have even wanted to be in a helping profession so she could give back what she had been given and help others.

If this account sounds familiar to you, it is because brilliant survivors – including survivor-professionals like she had become – are rising up all round the world. But while this description may sound optimistic, it is sadly open to new perils from unexpected quarters: professional complaints, the shadow side of treatment. In this chapter, I describe six types of complaints that tend to emerge out of these (or similar) circumstances.

1. A third-party complaint from a patient's alleged abuser
2. A third-party complaint after death
3. The patient retractor as complainant
4. The patient's complaint about the saviour, the cold mother and the terminator therapist
5. The next professional complainant
6. The criminal complaint
   a) The predatory therapist
   b) The tragic re-enactment

1. Third-party complaint from an alleged abuser

And then, out of the blue, the therapist received a complaint.

The patient's parents/neighbours/teachers/clerics wrote to the therapist's accrediting body saying the therapist must have planted false memories of bizarre abuse that could never have happened and had alienated their loved child from them.

The accrediting body (and this is almost all of them) felt forced to welcome this third-party complaint in its anxiety to 'protect the public'.

In other words, the culture of the organization was a fearful one in which a complaint raised fears of organizational reputational damage. It took months to determine the case (which one barrister said would have been thrown out of court within half an hour), and it was in the therapist's favour. The therapist, with no help from their accrediting body, had to contain the destabilized patient as well as fighting her case and dealing with her own anxieties (see Chapter 4). While the allegedly innocent family continued their attacks via social media, the therapist was bound to silence.

Additionally, most professional insurance companies who cover registrants of the various accrediting bodies do not protect their members from slander under their standard cover. The key advice from senior bodies was that clinicians should keep their silence, so as not to give such individuals or groups the 'oxygen of publicity'. Unlike a court experience, which would allow public vindication and damages, the private nature of the findings of the disciplinary panel does not aim for public social justice.

In 1996, Marjorie Orr, the pioneer creator of Accuracy about Abuse, wrote a major article on the 'Culture of Fear' in *Counselling News*. Marjorie Orr aided survivors and all working with them by pointing out presciently that the American false memory attacks on therapists would happen in the UK. In that period the main British therapy insurers and barrister considered false memory claims against therapists were not expected to have an effect, were rare in the UK and that there was no legal duty of care to parents of an adult child with capacity. Marjorie Orr was writing following the infamous Holly Ramona case in the USA where the father sued the therapist in a third party complaint over his daughter's disclosure of abuse by him.

As Bowman and Mertz (1996, p. 637) pointed out, 'By permitting a third-party recovery, the legal system allowed her parent instead to obliterate her, to make her invisible, to infantilize her and to take away her opportunity to confront directly what she viewed as a denial of her own very personal truth.' However, we have followed the American position in which litigation has increased. With the closure of the American False Memory Syndrome Foundation in December 2019, it remains to be seen whether litigation lessens. The legal issues around third-party complaints are very complex. However, in ordinary circumstances, such third-party liability excludes the client's wishes and could harm survivors, therapists and society more than helping wrongly accused parents.

The patient received confirmation of her family's warnings that anyone who helped her would be punished. This made it hard for her to reveal some of the most unbearable aspects of her life and brought in an obstacle to the heart of the therapeutic process. The woman's attachment to her mental health professionals who supported her was being held against her and against her team. How could she bring more damage to them?

Only in small numbers of cases do we see both the therapist and patient receive adequate support and be able to continue in their roles. And only in small numbers of cases do the therapist and patient manage to continue their work.

2. A third-party complaint after death

Following a successful flight from abuse, the patient had been able to live a few years of her adult life in relative safety, aided by a couple of friends. She built up a small volunteer support group who helped her as well, despite her warning them they were putting themselves in danger. She said that her family told her they would destroy the reputation of all organizations, professionals and volunteers who helped her.

Like many survivors, our template patient suffered many health problems. After some years of struggling with ill health, she sadly died prematurely. As she was young, she had not made a will so the very people she wanted to escape from had access to her remaining belongings and personal diaries and records. Very few survivors and survivor organizations have taken on board this complex legal and ethical question. Although, with extreme trauma, we note curtailed lifespans, it is counter-intuitive for survivors to be writing their wills at a younger age than the rest of the population. Nevertheless, this needs to be thought about as, without it, allegedly abusive families receive the estate of their dead child and all the medical records.

After a period following her death, her allegedly innocent family/clerics/professionals/neighbours banded together, not to understand her life and trauma, but to attack and mock anyone who had helped her. In our templated case they made a formal complaint.

Earliest treatment providers said they did not want to be named. 'Innocent' relatives of the family and neighbours did not want to be named as witnesses out of fear of repercussions despite the importance of their evidence and the promise of protection. Doctors and surgeons did not want to be named, partly under the advice of their professional bodies. Insurance companies demanded silence.

Whilst eventually disciplinary bodies declared there was no case to answer, the situation was not over for the therapist. The allegedly innocent complainants were free to invite media feasts and continue to attack the acquitted therapist. Furthermore, the therapist had to consider the ethics of what could and could not be said about a patient who had died. Confidentiality is an intrinsic part of the therapeutic relationship whether the patient is alive or dead.

Additionally, there is the right of the patient to privacy after death.

Of course, there can be third-party complaints that are correct and we need thoughtful structures that can manage this. Professionals and Disciplinary Panels can hopefully learn to differentiate between biased or litigious complainants and a genuinely grieving family. To add to the complexity, sometimes, of course, abusive family members and others dissociate from their past actions and genuinely grieve.

3. The patient 'retractor' as complainant

Our patient, despite her gains in some elements of the life she had wanted (for example, career success) becomes increasingly worn down and dispirited by the struggle. Ill health, the attacks on her clinicians and other professionals she has become attached to and fear of attacks on new partners or children take their toll, and events that endorse the disinformation of the abusers bring more despair to the survivor. A new untrained member in a mental health team or a psychotherapist who has not specialized in this area can evoke fear and terror in the patient. Going through a new assessment, waiting to hear about funding – all this can feel too much. The patient's sense of hope diminishes, and her spirit grows weaker, exacerbated by concern for those she fears are in danger.

Her family had always told her she was trouble and anyone she spoke to would be in trouble. A dangerous sequence can therefore follow. Some alters (or 'personalities'), who slowly chose to disclose, now wished they had not and wished they had joined in with the more hidden abuser-identified parts. Those who were abuser-identified were often amnesic to the trauma that created them and had only good memories of the perpetrators. To regain the love of their abusing families, cult-loyal and victim alters are put under great pressure to make a complaint about their therapist or doctor. Sometimes, when life becomes too unbearable and hopes for a better life are lost, they finally give up and give in.

In some situations, they can become 'retractors', ferociously condemning those who had helped them. Insurance plays a worrying part here too with some companies paying out compensation money, against the wishes of the person complained about, because the organizations they represent want to 'move on' or are worried about reputational damage for the organization.

Working with internal perpetrator–loyal alter personalities is extremely difficult. Those who enter the field of working with victims of abuse might not feel able to work with internalized abusers. There is also a hard lesson to learn about the aetiology of criminal behaviour (Sinason, 2017). In *The Orpheus Project* (Sinason, 2022) I explore this particularly difficult problem through fiction. Just as the patient was betrayed by attachment figures who hurt her instead of protecting her, those who supported the patient may face betrayal.

4. The patient's complaint about the saviour, the cold mother and the terminator therapist

The patient goes to a therapist who has never done this kind of work before. They feel an affinity with each other, and the therapist feels she can learn, with supervision, how to manage this work. The therapist anxiously and avidly scans the internet, goes to conferences, reads books. While learning a lot, she is also deeply affected. She becomes identified and enmeshed with her patient and is overwhelmed by the emotional projections into her. She finds herself prescriptively and nervously warning the patient against certain outings or meeting certain people (ironically, this rather mimics the origin of psychoanalytic work when Freud told a patient not to go to a dance), and spends increasingly long hours protecting the patient outside their session times. The patient expresses gratitude and says she feels safe for the first time (the saviour).

Then something very different happens. The patient makes a complaint.

The complaint usually comes when the therapist, through taking on more such work, gaining extra supervision or through a combination of life events became (temporarily or permanently) unable to maintain the same level of involvement. Whilst initially the patient says she felt heard and received she later complained that was untrue and she felt enmeshed, controlled and intruded on. Indeed, all the resources that were initially provided for her are now complained about. This defence against loss and change tips the emotional response to the therapist and the patient changes from perceiving the therapist as a saviour to being intrusive and engulfing, or cold and abandoning. This further frightens the patient. The patient who reports such behaviours in their therapist often describes a familial scenario in which, if mother is not on your side, your life is in danger as another sibling is being favoured (the cold mother).

Ending therapy is the next most common complaint concerning the failure of the therapist in the patient's mind. Termination often comes after two particular stages in therapy. The first is when the therapist realized that the patient is still at risk when the therapist had entered this work feeling she was helping adult survivors whose abuse was in the past.

The second point of vulnerability came when she encountered, for the first time, a personality who identified with the alleged abusers. The therapist had no experience of working with victim-perpetrators. After sleepless nights and a breakdown of her immune system, the therapist became ill and stopped treatment. When she felt more equipped to work again, she did not feel she could face the patient and therefore treatment was ended in a clumsy way with the patient being told her therapist was ill and no further meeting could be provided (the terminator). In each of these scenarios, the patient makes a complaint out of fear for their own survival.

5. The next professional complainant

In this scenario, for whatever reason, the therapist had ended the work with the client. The ending could be poorly managed (as in the previous scenario) or even a well-prepared retirement with a long notice period (see Chapter 1).

It takes the patient a while to find an alternative therapist and go through all the hurdles that are in the way of gaining skilled and funded treatment. In addition, the patient must go through terrible fear and internal punishment for speaking out again.

However, after all such trials, the patient/client finds someone new they dare to trust again and are deeply satisfied with the new therapist. This person not only seems to understand the pain of the whole system and the appalling abuse they describe but also appears to understand and sympathize with the patient's grievance against her previous therapist. Indeed, the new therapist is so angry on behalf of the client that they offer to help the client in making a complaint or even to act as a witness.

Joan Golston (Pre-Conference Ethics Workshop, ISSTD, March 2018, Chicago), Adah Sachs (Chapter 1) and other experts in this field have highlighted the particular 'saviour' feelings a second therapist can feel when taking on the treatment of a new client who has suffered so much. Indeed, the claim of 'being a witness' springs from the new therapist witnessing the suffering of the patient and being affected by it. It is not, however, true: a witness is a person who was present during an offence being committed and can thus testify to their knowledge about a wrongdoing. While the patient's suffering is true, an offence committed by the previous therapist may not be true.

As the complex role of the new therapist becomes more understood, we hope it will become systemically easier to differentiate between appropriate complaints and enacted ones. The problem is not that the patient can unconsciously misdirect to the innocent first therapist the powerful affect of real abuse they have experienced, it is where the second therapist considers that it must all be true. A therapist is not a police officer or judge and jury and has to hold the significance of emotional truth which may or may not be distorted. Of course, there are worrying occasions where abuse by the previous therapist is investigated and found to be true and rightfully evokes concern in the second therapist. Abuse can vary from unintentional boundary breaks to criminal action. At the non-criminal end there are organizations which aid professionals who have problems with their boundaries such as The Centre for Boundary Studies (UK).

Both the first and second therapist's counter-transference can usefully indicate the nature of trauma to the patient (Johns, 2022) and it requires experienced supervision to navigate these difficult areas. In terms of the issues focused on in this chapter, however, it is where a second therapist is unable to keep to their therapeutic task that this issue rises.

6. The criminal complaint

This falls into two categories.

      a)   The predatory therapist
      b)   The tragic re-enactment

(a) The predatory therapist

The patient, having thought they had escaped from their family and past contacts, and with their dissociation protecting them from knowledge of different kinds of ongoing contact, feels a deep sense of relief at starting therapy with someone who really seems to understand. After years of submitting to orders, the patient does not notice the subtle ways in which the therapist is taking charge of their life. Community connections and liaison with other services are subtly and slowly discouraged as the therapist is providing everything that is needed. By the time sexual abuse happens many of the personalities consider it part of ordinary life, just as they had experienced previously, except this is often initially seen as 'love' by the patient or some of the personalities. This complaint, however rare, is devastating as it brings with it profound personal and institutional betrayal. It underlines the idea that authority is abusive and cannot be trusted and highlights the inequality of the relationship (Gabbard, 1989). To be hurt in the place where you sought and expected help can be more damaging than the original abuse, where sadistic and exploitative norms were accepted.

(b) The tragic re-enactment

The patient, having thought they had escaped from their family and past contacts and with their dissociation protecting them from knowledge of different kinds of ongoing contact, feels a deep sense of relief at starting therapy with someone who really seems to understand. But in some cases, the therapist's ability to really understand is based on the similarity between the patient's trauma to the therapist's own traumatic past. And in a subset of these cases, where the therapist's own trauma had not been fully processed, it could erupt and cause harm rather than good. The therapist might understand the patient only too well, feeling symbiotically twinned with her because of their own half-forgotten trauma which the work with this patient shockingly and suddenly opens. The therapist had no intention of causing harm to any patient and, moreover, had entered the field specifically to help others in gratitude to their own past therapy which allowed them, they felt, to step beyond their own trauma history to enable others to reclaim their lives. The therapist felt such pain for the patient's sexual disgust, self-injury and enforced celibacy, which they realized matched their own, that they fell into an illusion, which had never applied to any other patient, that they were providing sexual healing and love. However rare, such violations cause devastating consequences. Indeed, Pope and Vetter (1991) found that 80 per cent of those who had a sexual relationship with the therapist only after therapy had ended had nevertheless still been severely harmed. Inclusion of such issues in trauma training is important as well as enabling supervisors and training organizations to be aware of this. The erotic transference and counter-transference need to be properly included in all trainings.

Even now, researchers (Pope *et al*, 2021) found that 87 per cent of psychologists reported sexual attraction to a client, 63 per cent felt guilty about it and only 9 per cent reported any useful training on the issues and therefore did not understand sexual transference and counter-transference. Little has changed. Forty years ago, whilst awareness of sexual attraction towards a patient existed in some mental health professionals, it evoked so much guilt and discomfort that the psychological aspects and the 'ordinary' projections could not be discussed. That fear and discomfort was exacerbated by the lack of input by training bodies.

Conclusion

A prerequisite for Dissociative Identity Disorder (DID) is trauma at a young age (Fonagy and Target, 1995). This means it is largely a forensic condition with all the extra concerns outer reality brings into the internal world of psychotherapy (Sachs and Galton, 2008). Psychotherapists who feel equipped for dealing with victims of past abuse can feel undertrained when abuse is also current and crimes are being disclosed. In the absence of supportive community teams and vulnerable victim-coordinators, the therapist can feel extremely vulnerable.

However, there is not only the live issue of crime but also the level of betrayal and shame that is experienced by the patient. There are other individuals who suffer gross trauma without developing a DID. The significant extra ingredient is betrayal coming from the experiences that lead to a disorganized attachment. Liotti (1992) was one of the first to apply understanding of this attachment pattern to dissociation. The nature of this attachment has been linked to lethal attachment (Sinason, 1990), internalized death wishes (Sinason, 1992) and infanticidal attachment (Kahr, 2007) and further developed by Sachs (2008, 2011, 2013, 2017). In other words, there has been trauma linked to an attachment figure. This makes personal betrayal and the perception of personal betrayal an extremely heightened expectancy.

Greater understanding is important but of course it cannot solve everything. Trauma-informed psychotherapy is relational, and this makes it a powerful crucible for change and hope, but it also houses inevitable re-enactments and damage.

A woman in treatment for 13 years said to her therapist, 'I am just beginning to think I might be able to trust you. You could have been nice to me all these years in the hope of suddenly tricking me and abusing me.' This is the true level of betrayal against which remarkable work is accomplished. Many patients who come from a DID and ritual abuse background say to their therapist, 'My family have told me that anyone I tell, especially a professional, will be attacked as well as me for speaking out.' Their own attachment needs are held against them (Badouk Epstein et al, 1996). This is what they have been told by their abusers. The tragedy is, without further understanding and change, there is still truth in it.

We hope the courage of therapist and patient is supported and that understandings from this book will inform practice. Paying attention to complaints that come from the six key categories provided could potentially allow treatment to continue without the damaging disruptions currently occurring.

Notes

1.   This condition is largely a survival mechanism to hide overwhelming abuse from an attachment figure at a young age. The child cannot fight or flee physically but can leap into another part of their mind so creating an alter-personality, or self-state or part who is protected by an amnesic wall from knowing what has happened.

PART II

HISTORICAL PERSPECTIVE

CHAPTER 6

Filing psychoanalytical complaints: from verbal assaults to the crushing of the larynx

Brett Kahr

False allegations and justifiable lawsuits

In my experience, the very vast majority of mental health professionals who practise in the twenty-first century comport themselves with tremendous compassion, kindness, professionalism, and honourability. Most psychological workers – whether psychiatrists, psychotherapists, psychologists, counsellors, social workers, creative arts therapists, or psychoanalysts – appreciate only too clearly how much our patients will already have suffered throughout their infancies and childhoods. Consequently, we all endeavour to treat our patients with as much humanity as possible. And in most cases, we do so with great concern and, ultimately, efficacy.

Sadly, at times, some of our colleagues will perpetrate regrettable acts of cruelty by exploiting or abusing patients, often engaging in sexual relationships with vulnerable individuals. These breaches of professional ethics occur very infrequently indeed, but, alas, we all know of such instances. Fortunately, our membership bodies have created ethics committees, designed to monitor our behaviour and to champion the highest standards of practice. And, nowadays, if a patient or client should file a formal complaint against a registered mental health practitioner, the relevant ethics committee will launch an official investigation, thus ensuring that the patient will be heard properly.

I recently spoke to the Chief Executive Officer of one of the United

Kingdom's leading mental health organizations, which serves as the registration body for thousands of psychologically trained clinicians. It pleases me to report that this high-ranking colleague confirmed that fewer than *one per cent* of registered members will ever receive a formal complaint from a patient. Of course, certain patients or clients might be too frightened to register a formal complaint; hence, this figure may not be fully accurate. But, at least according to the official statistics of this noted membership body, over *ninety-nine per cent* of clinical practitioners do comport themselves in a truly meticulous manner and will never become the subject of an official accusation. Of the very small percentage of colleagues who *do* receive a complaint, only an extremely tiny handful will ever be removed from the membership roster, owing to the fact that many complaints from patients cannot always be justified, and some of those complaints might well be an expression of negative transference or, indeed, a sign of unconscious retaliation against ancient parental figures who had once abused their children.

Indeed, some complaints from patients can readily be disproven and dismissed as false allegations. Perhaps most famously, back in 1975, a woman in Australia endured a dreadful trauma when a man entered her home and sexually molested her. The victim eventually filed a formal complaint, identifying the perpetrator as the noted Australian psychologist, Dr Donald Thomson, a Senior Lecturer at Monash University in Melbourne. It soon emerged, however, that Dr Thomson had the very best of alibis as he happened to be speaking *live* on television, on the Australian Broadcasting Corporation, at the time of this abusive episode; and it seems that the victim happened to remember only *his* name and face, at which she stared on the television screen while her assailant attacked her (Baddeley, 1982, 2004). Thus, complaints may, in certain instances, be unjustified and aimed incorrectly at an innocent mental health worker.

But, sometimes, alas, complaints against psychological practitioners can be quite accurate. One need but recall the painful case of Evelyn Walker, a woman from San Diego, California, who, back in the 1970s, underwent psychoanalytical treatment with the highly accomplished physician and psychoanalyst, Dr Zane Dribin Parzen, one of the former trainees of the esteemed Professor Heinz Kohut at the Chicago Institute of Psychoanalysis in Chicago, Illinois. Over the course of treatment, Dr Parzen seduced this patient on the psychoanalytical couch on many occasions, and, after Mrs Walker filed a complaint, a court hearing ensued, which resulted in a huge financial settlement of some $4,600,000 and, moreover, in the suspension of Dr Parzen's medical licence (Walker and Young, 1986) and his resignation from membership in the American Psychoanalytic Association (Anonymous, 1981).

The story of Zane Parzen stands out as one of the first legal cases against a practising psychoanalyst. Fortunately, nowadays, professional ethics committees and law firms regularly provide thorough and vigilant assessments of complaints by patients in order to achieve the most honourable of outcomes. But, back in the early days of psychoanalytical practice, prior to the formalization of the selection standards of candidates and the implementation of highly structured curricula of modern training programmes, and long before the creation of ethics committees or professional standards committees (which rarely existed prior to the Second World War), we must wonder how psychoanalytical patients actually expressed any complaints against their treating therapists, and how those clinicians would thus have responded?

Often, early Freudian analysands would express their rage in a private, verbal manner, within the confidential confines of the consulting room. Perhaps most dramatically, one of Professor Sigmund Freud's (1918) patients, Sergéi Konstantínovich Pankéev, better known as the 'Wolf Man' (or, in the original German, as 'Der Wolfsmann'), referred rather anti-Semitically to the father of Viennese psychoanalysis as a 'Jüdischer Schwindler' (Freud, 1910a, p. 214), namely, a 'Jewish swindler'. As Freud (1910b, p. 138) confessed in a letter to his Hungarian colleague, Dr Sándor Ferenczi, this very troubled patient, Pankéev, had even threatened to sodomize his psychoanalyst and 'shit on my head'.[1] Needless to say, we cannot provide a legally binding assessment of the nature of the Wolf Man's complaints and threats against Freud. It might well be the case that the patient terrorized Freud as a response to a certain type of unethical, abusive behaviour, but, likewise, it could well be that, owing to the patient's very fragile and traumatized history, the Wolf Man's desire to rape Freud and to defecate upon him may have represented a means of conveying the full nature of the patient's early history in a transferential form.

Thus, certain patients would 'file' complaints through the expression of rage within the consulting room. But other patients would convey their fury in a far more deadly manner.

The horrid crime of Rudolf Hug

In the small hours of the morning of 9 September 1924, a young Austrian man named Rudolf Otto Hug broke into the apartment of the esteemed 53-year-old psychoanalyst, Dr Hermine von Hug-Hellmuth, in Vienna, and murdered her by crushing her larynx, breaking her ribs, and smashing her skull (Deutsch, 1973). Herr Hug then stole some 2,600,000 Kronen from this dead woman as well as a gold watch (MacLean and Rappen, 1991).

Rudolf Hug, known more informally as 'Rolf', had many reasons to be angry. He became orphaned at the very young age of nine years after his mother had died from tuberculosis. He then attempted suicide sometime thereafter and spent a period in an institution for delinquent adolescents. But, in addition to these very understandable sources of aggression, Herr Hug had at least one other reason to be rageful. His mother's sister, Dr Hermine von Hug-Hellmuth, one of the very first Viennese practitioners of child psychoanalysis, decided that her nephew should undergo treatment, and she encouraged him to lie upon her very own couch. Thus, Dr von Hug-Hellmuth actually psychoanalyzed her young nephew, thereby exposing his very private world of sexual and aggressive thoughts and fantasies.

Quite a number of the early psychoanalysts did, indeed, treat their own biological relatives, not least Professor Sigmund Freud, who subjected his youngest daughter, Anna Freud, to a lengthy period of personal analysis (Roazen, 1969). But Anna Freud never murdered her father. Evidently, she had enjoyed a more securely attached childhood and she remained a lifelong fan of Sigmund Freud. However, Rudolf Hug, by contrast, had already endured immense loss and trauma and bereavement; hence, when his aunt subjected him to psychoanalysis and would have encouraged him to reveal his most intimate secrets, he became rageful and then killed her in an extremely vicious manner.

Needless to say, this episode in the early history of psychoanalysis proved most traumatizing for all concerned. Hermine von Hug-Hellmuth lost her life. Rudolf Hug spent many years in prison. And the members of the psychoanalytical community of Vienna – all close disciples of Sigmund Freud – endured much fear and terror, knowing that this sort of scandal would damage the reputation of their work. Indeed, Herr Hug actually endeavoured to sue the psychoanalysts of Vienna as he felt that he had suffered at their hands. Dr Felix Deutsch, who served for many years as Sigmund Freud's *Leibarzt* – personal physician – had to hire a private detective to protect his wife, Dr Helene Deutsch (1973) Indeed, Freud, one of von Hug-Hellmuth's close colleagues, as Rudolf Hug had begun to stalk her.

Nowadays, in the twenty-first century, I very much doubt that any child psychoanalyst would treat his or her own nephew. This would be regarded as unethical by every single professional organization. An aunt or an uncle might recommend a trusted fellow professional to provide psychotherapy or psychoanalysis, but none of our colleagues would undertake such treatment himself or herself. Indeed, if Hermine von Hug-Hellmuth did psychoanalyze her nephew today, he would have had every right to file a formal complaint with the ethics committee of the Wiener Psychoanalytische Vereinigung, namely, the Vienna Psycho-Analytical Society. If that young man had done so, by expressing his resentment in words rather than actions, von Hug-Hellmuth might have enjoyed a much longer life and could well have made many more important contributions to the study of child mental health. Thankfully, the case of Rudolf Hug has proved quite a rarity in the history of psychoanalysis, as few other colleagues endured torture and murder by their analysands.

How did patients handle angry feelings back in the old days, before the implementation of formal complaints procedures? How did the psychoanalysts themselves process their own anger and aggression towards their more troubled and troubling patients?

In the pages which follow, we shall endeavour to explore this hitherto unexamined area of clinical practice during the foundational decades of the modern mental health profession, in the hope that such an historical investigation will help to remind us of the potential for toxicity in the intimate psychoanalytical relationship, and with the intention that we might, today, continue to learn from some of the challenges and struggles and, indeed, formal errors of our professional ancestors.

Posthumous complaints

During the early days of psychoanalysis, most complaints against practitioners would not be filed in courts and most of the analysands refrained from enacting their murderous feelings (whether justified or unjustified). A very large percentage 'filed' their complaints through gossip, insulting their psychoanalysts in conversation or writing, often decades after the treatment had ended. Sometimes, colleagues, too, would 'file' complaints through gossip, years later, deeply vexed and concerned by the behaviour of some of their one-time fellow practitioners.

Dr Wilhelm Stekel, one of Freud's very first disciples, proved to be a most dedicated, creative, and prolific researcher (for example, Stekel, 1909, 1910, 1911). Nevertheless, in the *Behandlungsraum* – namely, the consulting room – he perpetrated many acts of a dubious nature while communicating with his analysands. For instance, while treating Dr Fritz Wittels, an aspiring psychoanalyst in his own right, Stekel would, at times, encourage Wittels to lie upon the traditional psychoanalytical couch, but, on other occasions, he would take him on walks through 'snowfields scantily lit' (Wittels, 1992, p. 62) – often during the night – accompanied by Stekel's police dog, whose canine behaviour would often become far more the focus of Stekel's attention than the patient himself. Stekel not only failed to offer a consistent physical setting for Wittels but he often violated confidentiality by revealing details about his other patients (Wittels, 1992). Unsurprisingly, Fritz Wittels came to regard his analysis with Wilhelm Stekel as very unsatisfactory, as did many of his other analysands; indeed, Wittels seemed hardly surprised to discover that Stekel's treatments often lasted for only a very short period of time indeed (cf. Wittels, 1995). Stekel died in 1940, and Wittels passed away one decade later in 1950. These allegations did not appear in print until 1992; hence, one might consider Wittels's complaints as posthumous filings.

Stekel vexed not only his patient Wittels, but many other individuals as well. Throughout his long psychoanalytical career, he perpetrated many other acts of boundary-breaching. For instance, Stekel examined the genitals of one of his male patients who struggled with penile impotency, in an effort to see whether this man could become erect at that moment. According to Dr Edoardo Weiss – one of the pioneers of psychoanalysis in Italy – Stekel could be 'sexual with patients' (quoted in Roazen, 2005, p. 58). In later years, after Stekel emigrated to Great Britain, he treated an English patient, Dr Mary Capes, who reported that in the midst of her psychotherapeutic sessions, this émigré analyst would often play the piano (Stanton, 1988). Apparently, Stekel even requested that one of his male patients, the young physician, Dr Martin James (1997), should administer an enema to him.

Although Wilhelm Stekel had worked loyally in the early days to support the psychoanalytical movement and had provided some very impressive insights into the understanding of dreams (for example Stekel, 1909, 1911), which remain of clinical relevance to this day, these breaches of what has since become known as classical psychoanalytical technique, contributed to Freud's sense of irritation. It came as no surprise that, in spite of his early regard and affection for Stekel, Freud (1914, p. 264) eventually came to dismiss him as little more than a 'pig'. Indeed, Freud ultimately confessed to Wittels, 'I have committed two crimes in my life; I called attention to cocaine and I introduced Stekel to psychoanalysis.'[2] (quoted in Wittels, 1992, p. 67). Freud even came to refer to deviant forms of clinical practice as 'the non-Stekel brand' (Wittels, 1992, p. 68).

Fortunately, the vast majority of the early Viennese psychoanalysts did not examine the genitalia of their patients or request the administration of an enema or play the piano in the middle of treatment sessions. But many did violate confidentiality, engage in social activities with patients, reveal personal information, and so forth (Roazen, 1995; Kahr, 1999, 2022). Thus, we must wonder how on earth did such breaches of traditional professionalism occur and what options, if any, apart from gossip and murder, did a patient have when concerned about the behaviour of the treating clinician?

The case of Wilhelm Reich

Although, nowadays, the mental health profession boasts no shortage of intensive training programmes of every shape and size – whether certificates, diplomas, bachelor's degrees, master's degrees, and doctoral degrees, as well as postdoctoral intensive programmes, across many countries worldwide – prior to the 1920s formal psychotherapeutic or psychoanalytical training simply did not exist. According to Dr Wilhelm Reich, a young Austrian physician who joined the Freudian movement during that time, very few practitioners spoke about the specificities of clinical practice in a detailed manner. As Reich (1942, p. 29) explained, 'There were hardly any discussions of psychoanalytic technique, a lack which I felt very keenly in my work with patients. There was neither a training institute nor an organized curriculum. The counsel to be had from older colleagues was meager. "Just go on analyzing patiently," they would say, "It'll come." What would come, and how, one did not quite know.'[3].

Keen to enhance the depth and the reputation of clinical practice, Reich established his very own technical seminar for some of his younger fellow colleagues within the Vienna psychoanalytical community. As these up-and-coming practitioners hungered for more detailed clinical education and supervision, Reich's seminar proved quite popular, and one of the attendees, Grete Lehner (later Professor Grete Bibring), recalled that the meetings would often last until one o'clock in the morning (Sharaf, 1971a).[4]

Not only would Wilhelm Reich complain about the lack of a more substantial training in Vienna in the 1920s, but other psychoanalytical workers would do so as well. For example, the American psychiatrist, Dr Roy Grinker – psychoanalyzed by Freud himself – moaned about the paucity of training resources in Chicago, Illinois, during the 1930s. As Grinker (1985, p. 11) recalled, 'The teaching was minimal, terminating in a brief verbal examination and subsequent acceptance by the psychoanalytic establishment.' Essentially, Grinker described the training experience as little more than 'a period of self-development'.

When considering Wilhelm Reich's sense of discontent with the clinical practice of psychoanalysis back in the 1920s, one must wonder about the impact of his own disappointing experiences of being an analysand. His first psychoanalyst, Dr Isidor Sadger, maintained such loose professional boundaries that, after he finished working with Reich, he then began to treat Reich's close friend (and future lover), Lia Laszky, as a patient, and, on one occasion, he insisted upon fitting Fräulein Laszky with a diaphragm, which he inserted into her body mid-session (Sharaf, 1971c). Apparently, Reich revealed that several psychoanalysts in the early days would even touch their patients' genitalia (Sharaf, 1983), although it remains unclear whether they did so as part of a physical examination or due to sexually charged reasons.

Reich ultimately underwent a second analysis with Dr Paul Federn, known for eating food in sessions (Roazen, 1975). In consequence, this psychoanalytical experience proved unsatisfactory and did not last very long at all (Sharaf, 1971b).

In view of having undergone treatment from Sadger and Federn, neither of whom preserved the boundaries of neutrality nor devoted themselves to a complete focus on the patient, it might be of little surprise to know that, during one of his analyses (very probably with Sadger),

Reich managed to sneak a fellow medical student into the consulting room before the start of the session and hid him underneath the couch so that this young man could actually overhear a private psychoanalytical consultation. Decades later, Reich revealed to his young apprentice, Myron Sharaf, that Freud had come to learn about this episode and that, 'Freud was very angry when he heard about it' (quoted in Reich, 1948, p. 117). At least Sigmund Freud had the capacity to speak out against boundary violations even if he helped – however unwittingly – to perpetrate them himself (Kahr, 1999, 2022).

Perhaps in view of these early blurry boundary experiences, Wilhelm Reich ultimately became the pioneer of integrating psychoanalysis with the physical touching of his patients in an effort to help them to relax their muscles, thus prompting the development of a whole welter of body psychotherapies (for example, Geib, 1998; Smith, 1998a, 1998b; Farrell, 2006; Totton, 2020). For instance, we know that, at least as early as 1938, Reich would treat patients in various states of undress. Ola Raknes, a male Norwegian psychoanalyst, would attend consultations fully nude; and his female counterparts would undergo psychodynamically orientated body work dressed in their brassieres and panties (Sharaf, 1972).

But, moreover, such blurry boundaries impacted upon Reich as a clinician in other ways, no doubt through an unconscious identification with the lack of clarity perpetrated by his own personal psychoanalysts years previously. Indeed, during the 1950s, Reich treated a young man (and future psychologist), the aforementioned Myron Sharaf. At some point, circa 1953, Sharaf's wife – Grethe Hoff – who had, herself, undergone treatment from Reich, eventually consulted him about a medical matter, and, in due course, Dr Reich and Mrs Sharaf embarked upon an affair. Reich telephoned Sharaf – his patient – to inform him of this situation. In due course, the marriage exploded as a result of Reich's 'reckless action' (Sharaf, 1983, p. 30). As Myron Sharaf confessed decades later, he experienced a great deal of 'hurt and betrayal at the hands of Grethe and, especially, of Reich' (Sharaf, 1983, p. 30). Indeed, he felt 'doubly betrayed' (Sharaf, 1983, p. 431). In view of the fact that Reich's own psychoanalyst, Isidor Sadger, had treated Reich's one-time girlfriend and then fitted her with a diaphragm, such infractions seem hardly surprising.

Blurry boundaries could also manifest themselves in other ways in Reich's practice. In 1945, one of Reich's patients – a woman called Gladys Meyer – reminisced about how, during childhood, a boy had once threatened her with a knife. Shockingly, Reich, then practising in the American State of Maine, grabbed a pair of deer antlers and pointed this sharp object at his patient, mid-free association, ostensibly in an effort to provoke more reminiscences of the original trauma. This undisciplined, indeed, unethical action, frightened Gladys Meyer, who became quite scared and then jumped off of the couch (Sharaf, 1971d).

Thus, the story of Wilhelm Reich – encapsulated in an extremely brief manner – underscores how, during the very early days of this profession, even those keen to enhance the understanding of psychoanalytical technique had not sufficiently internalized clear boundaries. Consequently, many of the pioneering practitioners, in spite of their brilliance, would sometimes engage with patients in a complex and unprofessional style, thus providing the bedrock for the sorts of behaviours which, in subsequent decades, would become known, more formally, as unethical.

The growth of the ethics committee

Fortunately, as psychoanalysis began to develop and expand beyond the confines of Freud's consulting room, his growing circle of disciples became increasingly professionalized. So, in spite of the fact that the early practitioners did not undergo any *formal* training *per se*, by the 1920s, psychoanalytical institutes had begun to develop in Berlin, in Vienna, and in London (for example, Freud, 1924b; Freud and Freud, 1924; cf. Jones, 1957; Deutsch, 1973; Sterba, 1982; Roazen, 1985), each requiring not only admissions interviews for prospective candidates but, also, proper coursework and supervision of trainees, alongside their own experience of in-depth personal psychoanalysis.

For instance, in 1926, the Training Committee of the Institute of Psycho-Analysis in London implemented a requirement that all candidates must attend for supervision with at least one of three specific senior practitioners, namely, Dr Edward Glover, Dr Ernest Jones, or Dr John Rickman (Training Ctte Minutes: 24.3.1926–29.10.1945, 1926–1945). Not long thereafter, in 1928, this same committee insisted that all trainee psychoanalysts would now be required to submit regular reports about their patients, thus ensuring that clinicians would think about their analysands in detail and would permit their work to be scrutinized more carefully by their teachers.

Fortunately, in the post-World War II era – after the death of Sigmund Freud – the field of psychoanalysis had, by that point, become sufficiently well established and, also, reasonably prominent in certain circles that various organizations began, for the very first time, to implement the creation of formal ethics committees and professional standards committees, especially the American Psychoanalytic Association, which provided a very important role model for other organizations worldwide.

The post-war issues of the Bulletin of the *American Psychoanalytic Association* reveal that this growing membership body had constructed an increasing welter of committees which examined and imposed training guidelines and ethical requirements with much vigilance. For instance, the American Psychoanalytic Association had inaugurated a Board of Professional Standards, consisting of senior clinicians from each of its component societies and institutes, which became a veritable "watchdog" (Anonymous, 1948, p. 5) for American psychoanalysis. Indeed, even as early as 1948, the American Psychoanalytic Association had no difficulty boasting that, as an institution, it maintained standards "at so high a level" (Anonymous, 1948, p. 10). Not long thereafter, during his tenure as President of the American Psychoanalytic Association, Dr. William Menninger (1948, p. 1) – the brother of the noted clinician Dr. Karl Menninger, and a psychiatrist-psychoanalyst in his own right – proposed that this increasingly large national organisation should establish a *"certification board for psychoanalysis"* which would not only maintain standards of practice but would, also, unify those standards across different institutions and states.

Over time, this growing investment in the creation of high ethical principles developed profoundly, worldwide. Indeed, applicants would be required to undertake more training prior to the commencement of their formal psychoanalytical candidacies, and qualified practitioners would need to receive continuing professional education and would have to adhere to a detailed code of ethics. Consequently, members of the psychoanalytical communities would no longer be permitted to eat breakfast or dinner in the middle of sessions, or to marry their patients or, indeed, to examine their genitalia. As these post-war recommendations became implemented, the discipline had, at last, become increasingly professionalized and, therefore, much more efficacious and sterling than ever before.

Of course, even with the insistence upon the most intense of training and upon the most vigilant of professional standards, contemporary practitioners do still engage from time to time in a wide range of ethical breaches, as in the case of the American psychoanalyst, Dr Zane Parzen – to whom I have already referred – a physician and psychoanalyst who had embarked upon a sexual affair with one of his patients, Evelyn Walker. In consequence, Mrs Walker filed a lawsuit against Dr Parzen, who ultimately had to cease practice entirely (Walker and Young, 1986). Of course, one need not engage in sex with an analysand in order to breach ethics. In 1988, Francis Lederer, son of the wealthy Anne Lederer, sued his mother's long-standing psychoanalyst, Professor George Pollock – a sometime President of the American Psychiatric Association and, indeed, one of the most noted psychiatrists and psychoanalysts in the world – for having extorted approximately $5,000,000 from his mother's foundation, the Anne P. Lederer Research Institute, for his own purposes (Kirsner, 2000). Thus, infractions of ethical codes can manifest themselves in many forms indeed.

But, even if one adheres to all the codes appropriately and fails to breach any ethical rules, one might still comport oneself in a perfectly legal, though very *unpleasant* manner. Many years ago, the esteemed British psychoanalyst, Dr Brendan MacCarthy, told me a very shocking story about one of his long-standing, senior colleagues. Apparently, this man, whom we shall refer to as 'Dr X', had treated a young trainee in psychoanalysis over a period of more than ten years on a five-times-weekly basis. Upon the completion of the patient's formal training and upon his qualification as a psychoanalyst in his own right, this person prepared to terminate his long-standing treatment with Dr X and at the end of the final session of this lengthy, emotional process, the patient extended his hand for a shake. Dr X who regarded himself as a highly orthodox practitioner who would never blur a boundary, refused to shake the patient's hand as a farewell gesture. Although no one can arrest a psychoanalyst or remove a psychoanalyst from a published roster for having refused to shake a patient's hand (especially if such a request had occurred amid the Covid-19 pandemic), the patient felt extremely hurt and betrayed, and then confessed to Dr MacCarthy that Dr X's prissy unwillingness to touch hands actually spoiled his memories of their decade-long collaboration. The patient of Dr X never filed a formal complaint, but this person certainly did 'complain' in private conversations, no doubt to many other colleagues in addition to Brendan MacCarthy.

The unconscious transmission of ethical blurriness

When a contemporary psychoanalyst, such as Dr Zane Parzen, violates basic ethical practice by engaging in sexual relations with a patient, one can readily dismiss such a person as a troubled, irresponsible, even cruel, clinician, who remains a shunned outlier within the profession – a true criminal rarity. We have very little documentation about the inner world and early history of Zane Parzen, therefore, we cannot possibly offer a reliable comment as to why this man engaged in such activities. And we have no public information or archival data about his own experiences of psychoanalytical training which may or may not have impacted upon his behaviours. But we do have some data about various better-known figures in the history of psychoanalysis who had perpetrated sexual offences.

Let us now consider the case of Marilyn Monroe, whose California-based psychoanalyst, Professor Ralph Greenson, invited this iconic Hollywood star to move into his private home and to dine regularly with the members of his family. The majority of clinical psychotherapeutic practitioners do not offer bedrooms to patients, but Greenson did so, in part, perhaps, due to his concern that Miss Monroe – a fragile, publicly exposed film star – had little support structure in her life but, partly, one must suspect, due to Greenson's own sense of arousal at housing a beautiful woman whom many regarded as the most attractive and most alluring female on the planet at that moment in time (Greenson, 1978b; Freeman, 1992; Spoto, 1993). The case of Marilyn Monroe has generated immense controversy, and we may never be certain why Ralph Greenson violated so many traditional professional boundaries. But we have come to learn much more about Ralph Greenson's son, Daniel Greenson, who qualified as a physician and as a psychoanalyst in later life, having followed in his father's footsteps. Dr Daniel Greenson eventually rose to the rank of Training and Supervising Analyst at the well-regarded San Francisco Psychoanalytic Institute. Yet, having grown up in the home of his father – a psychoanalyst who had invited a sexy patient to live with the family – it may come as no surprise that Daniel Greenson, the son, eventually engaged in sexual boundary violations with one of his own patients and, ultimately, lost his hard-earned medical licence (Miller, 2014). Although we have little knowledge of the nature of Daniel Greenson's state of mind, one cannot help but wonder to what extent the son had identified with his father's questionable practices of turning the home into a consulting room for a sexy woman and, likewise, transforming the consulting room into a home.

The range of boundary violations across the history of psychoanalysis can be quite extreme and quite shocking, with Freud, one suspects, as the very best-behaved of all the clinicians. Nevertheless, Freud's occasional lack of clarity (for example, Kahr, 2022) could transmit rather rapidly across the generations. Let us not forget that Daniel Greenson had grown up in the home of Ralph Greenson (1978a), an American psychoanalyst who had studied under none other than Wilhelm Stekel, a man who played the piano during sessions, and who took his patients for night-time walks, and whom Freud had called a 'pig'. But let us also recall that Stekel (1948, p. 256) had undergone a very brief psychoanalysis, possibly 'not more than eight sessions', with none other than Freud himself (cf. Stekel, 1926, 1950; Bos and Groenendijk, 2007; Clark-Lowes, 2010). Dr Ernest Jones (1955, p. 7) discussed Stekel's psychoanalytical treatment with Professor Freud directly and, on the basis of those conversations, concluded that Stekel actually underwent a 'much more extensive' analysis. Whatever the length and depth of their clinical encounter, Freud and Stekel certainly crossed swords, and one cannot help but wonder what impact Freud's technique will have had upon Stekel and, consequently, upon those who followed in his wake.

Although we know little of the details of Stekel's very early experience of psychoanalysis with Freud, we can confirm that the relationship between these two pioneers ultimately exploded, and that Freud dismissed Stekel brusquely and criticized his former patient in his communications with their mutual colleague, Wittels, thus violating his obligation to ensure complete confidentiality (cf. Freud, 1923a, 1924a). Indeed, Freud actually lambasted Stekel – his former patient – as having 'unbearable manners',[5] and characterized him as full of 'treachery and ugly dishonesty',[6] – shocking statements of indiscretion regarding a former patient. One cannot help but wonder whether Freud's lack of pristine psychoanalytical neutrality with Stekel ultimately trickled down to Stekel's patient Greenson, who shared his home with Marilyn Monroe, and, subsequently, to Greenson's very own son who engaged in unethical sexual activity, resulting in the nullification of his medical licensure.

In view of the tremendously close links within Freud's tiny Jewish, Viennese, professional circles, one can understand even more fully how ethics and ideals became communicated only too readily. Appreciating the context of Freud's clinical work offers us a much greater understanding of the potential way in which his treatment of Wilhelm Stekel, for instance, followed by Stekel's treatment of Ralph Greenson, followed by Greenson's treatment of Marilyn Monroe, followed by Daniel Greenson's sexual boundary violations, can not only be transmitted forward but, also, traced backward across many generations. Therefore, although the so-called blurry boundaries perpetrated by Freud at a time when all psychoanalysts lacked any formal training may be considered rather mild and insignificant in the grand scheme of things, we must appreciate how, intergenerationally, even small acts of non-neutrality within the psychoanalytical sphere can, over time, impact upon subsequent practitioners in rather more ugly ways.

The best way to file a psychoanalytical complaint

Since Sigmund Freud (1896) first introduced the notion of psychoanalysis in the late nineteenth century, the psychological professions have grown at impressive speed and with increasing impact, not least as a consequence of the coronavirus pandemic. Fortunately, since the inception of the 'talking therapies', most psychotherapeutic and psychoanalytical practitioners have behaved in a truly ethical and honourable manner and have undertaken vital work to help prevent breakdowns and support fragile ego structures.

Regrettably, over the last century, a small number of psychoanalytical patients have complained about their psychoanalysts in a variety of fashions, ranging from gossip to murder. But fortunately, as our trainings have become more rigorous and more intense, as professional standards have increased, and as treatment has become more embedded as part of modern culture, the vast majority of clients or patients or analysands now participate in this process in a much more robust and appreciative manner. Of course, many patients will continue to express their infantile and childhood rage in the consulting room, often attacking the psychoanalyst or the psychotherapist in a verbal manner (for example, Kahr, 2020), and those patients who had already demonstrated criminality will even threaten the clinician in a more sinister fashion (for example, Kahr, 2004). Nevertheless, in spite of these challenges, most experienced mental health workers have found ways of containing such outbursts through a set of deep and rich conversations about the unconscious meanings of aggression in its many forms.

As we have learned from this brief historical investigation, complaints can arise at any time and can be enacted in a variety of fashions. Having reviewed the historical literature on this subject, I can confirm that the vast majority of complaints by patients had actually emerged in the pre-ethical era, before the establishment of longer training analyses and clearer ethical guidelines for practitioners. Many complaints developed through the unconscious intergenerational transmission of boundary violations across the decades; thus, by studying the history of our profession in greater detail, we now have the capacity to become more aware of the vulnerabilities of certain practitioners and to appreciate more fully the impact that such individuals must have had upon their trainees (cf. Kahr, 2021).

Mental health workers will occasionally engage in acts of unprofessionalism and even cruelty, such as the perpetration of sexual offences with one or more patients. In these instances (as in the case of Evelyn Walker), the analysand has the right to file a legal complaint. But it may well be that Sigmund Freud had already created the very best form of filing complaints, namely, the encouragement of patients to engage in the process of free association, thereby expressing the most violent emotions in words and thus minimizing the likelihood of behavioural enactments. Clearly, clinicians must invest more time in the study of negative transference, and in the toleration of our hatred in the countertransference (for example, Winnicott, 1949), so that we can both encourage our patients to be verbally angry and so that we can bear to hear the full extent of their early-life traumas. By doing so, we may well help our patients to complain in the most cathartic and, ultimately, curative manner.

Notes

1. The original German phrase reads, 'mir auf den Kopf scheißen' (Freud, 1910a, p. 214).
2. The original German sentence reads, 'Ich habe zwei Verbrechen begangen: daß ich auf das Cocain aufmerksam gemacht und daß ich den Stekel zur Psychoanalyse geführt habe' (quoted in Wittels, 1995, p. 179, n. 12).
3. This passage does not appear in the original 1927 German edition of Dr

Wilhelm Reich's book on the orgasm. In view of the fact that Reich still maintained close ties with the psychoanalytical community at that time, he certainly would never have criticized his elders in such a blunt fashion, not least as Professor Sigmund Freud had agreed to publish Reich's (1927) work under the banner of his very own Internationaler Psychoanalytischer Verlag [International Psycho-Analytical Press].

4.   Dr Myron Sharaf reported this information in his biography of Dr Wilhelm Reich but did not, alas, provide a detailed endnote as to which of his interviews with Professor Grete Bibring examined the early technical seminar which Reich facilitated in Vienna, Austria. On the basis of Sharaf's other citations of his conversations with Bibring, it seems most likely that she reminisced about his topic in the interview conducted on 10 April 1971 (Sharaf, 1971a).

5.   The original German phrase reads, 'unerträglichen Manieren' (Freud, 1923a, p. 346).

6.   The original German phrase reads, 'Hinterhältigkeit und unschöner Übervorteilung' (Freud, 1923a, p. 346).

Acknowledgements

I wish to express my deep thanks to Dr Adah Sachs and Dr Valerie Sinason for their kind invitation to contribute to this important edited volume.

CHAPTER 7

Reflections on a 25-year-old professional complaint

Leslie Ironside

It is now over 25 years since the allegation described in this chapter took place and the words and the aspect of the experience that are still most sharply seared into my memory are that the authorities 'did not feel I was a danger to my children'. This statement brought home to me in the most frightening form the possible and unthinkable extent of the consequences of the allegation: I might have been seen to be a danger to my children and therefore not be safe to live with them! How do you process such information? I am not sure you do! You live with it. It remains a trauma memory and impacts upon me in the here and now especially as I move into the next stage of my life and being a grandfather. This illustrates how an allegation so deeply and clearly impacts on one's personal life and personal sense of well-being. I know that this experience will be 'branded into my being' to my grave. I know that should another child make such an allegation, and this is perfectly possible given the nature of my work, that someone might well make assumptions and add the two experiences together in a way that could potentially be deeply destructive and have serious consequences.

But have I also learnt and grown from the experience? Yes, I do feel I have. I was fortunate to have very supportive family and friends, very supportive supervision, a very supportive professional network and personal analysis and this has stood me in good stead. This has meant that I do have 'belly knowledge' of an intrusive and difficult experience that can be contained, held and thought about and this has opened my eyes and informed my work with many people that have also had to manage, name and best process their own trauma memories. The process of writing the paper, having it accepted for publication, the act of 'going public' about the experience, have also been very helpful and I hope that the substance to the paper remains as relevant now as when it was first written.

'Serving two masters: a patient, a therapist, and an allegation of sexual abuse' (Ironside, 1998)

In this chapter, Leslie Ironside analyses a painful situation with which therapists are having to deal; when an abused child anticipates abuse in the therapy or distorts what is happening because he or she views all events through the prism of traumatic knowledge. Without polarizing or blaming, Leslie Ironside uses his training and experience to trace compassionately how such a situation can arise.

'We don't see things as they are, we see them as we are.'

Anaïs Nin

'It's often safer to be in chains than to be free.'

Franz Kafka

Therapists frequently have to struggle with the question of the veracity of what they are being told and to bear witness to the difficulties that patients might have as they, too, struggle with the question of the validity of their own memories. It is, though, important that therapists bear in mind the difference between patients' attempts to relate an event truthfully, that is, the struggle with memory, from the separate issue of what patients might want therapists to believe, that is, how patients might consciously or unconsciously alter what is communicated according to the present situation.

This issue takes on a particularly concrete dimension if a patient makes a false allegation of abuse, as a real, mutually witnessed event is transposed in the patient's mind to something quite different, and, at that point in time, the patient is clearly communicating a wish for something other than the actual experience to be believed. Such an event leads to important questions as regards the role of the therapist: how a therapist might be seen as an abuser, how this relates to the actual experience in the consulting room and in the patient's life history, and what light this might throw on a patient's pathology.

In his paper 'Observations on Transference-Love', Freud discussed the difficult technical issues of a patient falling in love with an analyst and the implications for technique and the strains that this can place upon the analytic relationship (Freud, 1915a). He concluded with the powerful thought that the therapeutic aim of psychoanalysis was 'to handle the most dangerous mental impulses and to obtain mastery over them for the sake of the patient' (p. 171).

Bion (1959, 1962b) later developed the concept of container and contained to describe the early infantile relationship between a mother and her child. Segal (1981) clearly summarizes how in this model:

> the infant's relation to his first object can be described as follows: when an infant has an intolerable anxiety, he deals with it by projecting it into his mother. The mother's response is to acknowledge the anxiety and do whatever is necessary to relieve the infant's distress. The infant's perception is that he has projected something intolerable into his object, but the object was capable of containing it and dealing with it. He can then reintroject not only his original anxiety but an anxiety modified by having been contained. He also introjects an object capable of containing and dealing with anxiety.

This concept of container and contained, and Winnicott's (1960a, b) subtly different concept of 'holding', are often also used to metaphorically describe the psychotherapist relationship with their patients and clearly links with Freud's dictum of obtaining mastery over dangerous mental impulses.

The situation involving a false allegation of sexual abuse by a therapist is a most testing example of attempting to contain (Bion), hold (Winnicott), or obtain mastery over (Freud) 'dangerous mental impulses' and raises crucial questions as regards the nature of memory and the relationship and difference between an individual's memory and what might best be described as the purpose of any particular communication.

In this chapter, I describe and explore what I have learnt from an experience with one particular child, Jim, in which an allegation led to a full diagnostic interview, a temporary breakdown in therapy, and, finally, a return to therapy. First, however, I would like to place this experience within a wider context through the exploration of work with three other patients in which allegations of various sorts were made but which did not lead to a belief within the professional network that there was any substance to them. In these three cases, the presenting material could then be thought through within the clinical setting and an attempt could be made to understand and 'obtain mastery' of (Freud) the material. This contrasts with the fourth case, which resulted in diagnostic interviews and a break in therapy – the correct course of action at that point, but one that served to mask rather than address the child's pathology.

Patient A: John

John was 13 at the time of referral but had the stature of a child many years his junior. One year prior to the referral, he had made an allegation that he had been abducted by a man and a woman and forced to have intercourse with the woman. No prosecution was ever made. A considerable amount of help had been offered to him and his family through the local family centre, and at the point of referral to me he was no longer in the house-bound state that he had been in for much of the previous year. At the initial meetings, he refused to see me alone, and so his mother remained in the room. He spoke of how he felt that he no longer trusted anybody except his family, and it soon transpired that there had been a long history of bullying and many difficulties in terms of separation prior to the alleged incident. Gradually, John settled enough to allow his mother to stay in the waiting room, which was very close to the consulting room, but both doors had to remain open. Unfortunately, during the first of the sessions when I was alone with him, he heard voices from another part of the building. John immediately became very anxious, and I, in a way that with hindsight might seem insensitive, asked if it would be helpful to shut the door. He now became overtly quite overwhelmed and tearful and wanted his mother. I asked his mother to come in.

Discussion

In his *Brazilian Lectures* (1990), Bion describes how in 'every consulting room there ought to be two rather frightened people: the patient and the psycho-analyst' (p. 5), but I think that John's fears go one step further than this. When his mother came back into the consulting room after the incident described, John was able to think about and discuss his fear; he also described how the voices had reminded him of the abductors and of how my then suggesting that the door should be closed linked me immediately with the gang and left him petrified and, of importance, of course, cut off from his mother. This immediately conjures up a picture of the need to consider complex emotional factors related to the infantile and primitive, as well as the present precipitating trauma. We can see from this example how in these perhaps extreme circumstances a patient can quickly see the therapist as an abuser. At the point of my suggesting shutting the door, John no longer seemed able to think symbolically; I seemed concretely, in Segal's terms, to become one of the abusing gang (Segal, 1991).

Patient B: Tony

Tony was 8 years old at the point of referral. Adshead (1994), in her review of the literature on false allegations of sexual abuse in childhood, states that in 96 per cent of such cases children do not deliberately set out to make trouble for adults. This did not seem to be the case with Tony, a boy who was causing immense anxiety to the professional network. His history was appalling. Both of his parents had died of drug overdoses, Tony himself discovering his mother's dead body one morning. His early childhood is likely to have been a haze of confusing images and awful events. He found it very difficult to relate to people; many would, of course, empathize with his story, but his coldness and violent behaviour would inevitably lead to a fiercely negative spiral of interaction. At the point of referral, there were immense concerns as regards his behaviour, a sense that he had never mourned for his parents and that he was finding it difficult to form meaningful relationships.

His attitude to therapy was, needless to say, very ambivalent, and I often felt that he would do all within his power to try to end the sessions. The professional network, though, remained steadfast in its opinion that Tony should continue in therapy. This was very difficult, and it was only due to immense effort and close communication between all the professionals involved that we managed to survive his attacks upon any commitment to form a therapeutic alliance with me and consequently to struggle with the dependency feelings that this would entail. I purposefully say 'we', as it was very much a group effort, with the escort who brought Tony being a very key figure in what was eventually felt to be a successful outcome to therapy.

The attacks were very forceful, going to the extent of his bruising himself and then making accusations that I had hit him. At times, I had to restrain him in the room, and, at times, the escort had to carry him physically into the room. He was also verbally very aggressive, though it was not so much what he said but the force with which he said things that made it so difficult to relate to him. He also said that he was going to tell his social worker that I had sexually abused him and then I would be locked up.

We always approached his behaviour as a communication of a frame of mind that needed to be understood, rather than to be acted upon in the sense of ending the sessions or formally investigating the allegations. This began to pay dividends, as I think he began to feel that his internal rage could be understood. It was, however, very difficult to maintain this frame of mind and not to feel overwhelmed by the thought that we were just cruelly and sadistically punishing him further. Then in one particular session, Tony greatly enlightened me, and his actions gave me the courage to continue the work. During the session, I had to deal with the most difficult attacks, both verbal and physical. Towards the end, he said that he was going to write me a letter. He had recently taken to writing, and, although this activity was often loaded with insults, I had seen it as a positive development in itself. (Interestingly, this coincided with the beginnings of some progress in his written work at school.) He quickly and secretly wrote something which he took with him and posted back through the letter box after the session ended. I had expected something similar to his other writings – 'Fuck off Ironside. I hate you' – but what he had written was, 'Dear Ironside ... I like you really ... Tony'. Needless to say, this greatly reinforced the importance of continuing the sessions despite the part of Tony that acted as a powerful saboteur almost destroying any hope of forming a close relationship, and I feel, giving a particularly dramatic exposition of the saying, 'He is his own worst enemy'.

Gradually, Tony allowed his foster parents to form a closer relationship with him, both physically and emotionally, and, again gradually, he began to form a more caring relationship with me in which he began to relate his life history, without re-traumatization.

Discussion

In the article 'Love and Death in the Transference: The Case of the Hungarian Poet Attila Jozsef', the author Mauro Mancia (1993) describes the equally powerful negative transference between Jozsef and his analyst which, as with Tony, was likely to have its origins in his infantile experience. Of most relevance to the theme of this chapter, however, are the following free associations, which he communicated in the form of blank verse.

I'll be lying ...

I'll mix truth with lies, I won't take it lying down ...
so I'll screw her up in her everyday life, outside analysis
I'll ruin her in her profession
I'll pass the word "by chance" that I've had it off with her ...
that way I'll get her to lick my arse
that was the relationship my mother got me into with her behaviour ...

This was written in 1936 just prior to his breaking off analysis. In December 1937 Attila Jozsef committed suicide at the age of 32, throwing himself under a train.

The subject, then, of false allegations of this malicious type is thus not a new one, although I think that the difference today is that such allegations can be thought about when working with a child of the tender age of 6 years who might or might not himself have been sexually abused. As in the case of Attila Jozsef and his awful death, my experience with Tony seemed also to indicate a very troubled person. He related to the outside world according to an internal phantasy of the 'everybody is my enemy' kind. Generally, his relationships were governed by a state of projective identification (Klein, 1946), dominated by a way of relating not with a person as separate from himself, with their own thoughts and feelings, but with this image projected into another person and then related to as though it belonged to that other person. The mechanism of projective identification has both developmental and defensive potential but this was a very rigid defensive position with the consequent confusion of ego boundaries and the formation of a relationship based on part objects that took a great deal of time to work through with Tony. He was referred in the first place because of concerns as regards the mourning process, and, as John Steiner (1993) argues in *Psychic Retreats*, it is in the process of mourning that the deep-rooted issues involved in projective identification can be resolved.

Without entering into a debate as to how one measures successful therapeutic outcome (cf. Boston and Lush, 1994), there was a general consensus in the network that Tony benefited a great deal from therapy. The key factor in this success seemed to be the close co-operation and mutual support that existed within the network. It was a system that was able to bear the allegations and remained convinced that these were manifestations of psychic distress and not matters that needed to be acted upon, other than ensuring that there was supportive professional contact at all times and an overt recognition of the destructive way in which Tony could relate. This theme of the importance of good communication within the professional network and awareness of processes such as destructive splitting is something that is so often stressed in the literature – for example, Reder and Duncan (1993), Bentovim (1992) and Sinason (1994).

Patient C: Peter

Peter was referred because of unmanageable behaviour that was beginning to threaten seriously his adoptive placement. He was a boy who had been multiply abused prior to his being taken into care, and he brought to therapy all the vexed issues associated with working with children who have been abused (cf. Boston and Szur, 1983; Szur and Miller, 1992). Again, there was within the professional network the very close communication that is so necessary in this type of work. Peter would be very flamboyant in his acting out and, in a tragicomic way, would call out the window that I was sexually abusing him, telling his escort and his social worker a similar story.

Discussion

On a conscious level he was alleging abuse, but in a way that meant that the allegations would not be taken seriously. This way of relating did give me, as the therapist, some insight into his internal world and into the relationships of his internal objects, but I would like to concentrate here on the issue of the allegations, which were not viewed by the network as warranting an investigation of the immediate events but, rather, were taken seriously and seen as a communication of a frame of mind that was particularly relevant in terms of this boy's life history.

This way of behaving must also be viewed in a wider context, in that this kind of behaviour, like the humourless behaviour exemplified by Tony, may be exhibited by children who have not been abused. Colleagues in both social work and teaching speak of observing this behaviour both with children they see professionally and with a wide spectrum of children not confined to those in which there is a suggestion of abuse. The knowledge of child sexual abuse is now abroad in the playground. This is the negative side of the more positive movement to raise public awareness and is an area of great concern at present, as professionals struggle to deal with the malicious allegations of abuse whilst recognizing that professional abuse does occur. There are side effects to increased public awareness of sexual abuse, one of which is how the conscious and unconscious anxieties brought about through such knowledge are borne both by children and by adults.

Allegation and investigation: Patient D

In contrast to the above three patients, Patient D made an allegation that was felt to warrant a full investigation. This experience highlights the struggle to ensure that a child is being adequately protected – professional abuse does take place – while paying attention to the very damaging impact of a false accusation upon a professional, and, indeed, upon the course of a child's therapy.

Jim, a 4-year-old who had been multiply abused, including incidents of brutal sexual abuse, made an allegation to his foster mother, following the first session after an Easter break, that I had given him some medication that had made him sleepy and that I had then 'played' with his penis. It was an allegation that had to be pursued in terms of child protection; a case conference was held, and a full diagnostic interview involving the police and social workers was completed. As a result of this allegation, not only was Jim's own therapy threatened but my own professional and personal life was placed under scrutiny and threat.

As Attila Jozsef wrote:

so I'll screw her up in her everyday life, outside analysis
I'll ruin her profession.

Such an issue blurs the boundary between the personal and professional life of the therapist.

The context

I saw Jim once weekly in my consulting room at home. This is a situation that must rank high in terms of (1) the possibility of an allegation being made, because of such a child's heightened feelings of vulnerability at being alone with an adult, and (2) providing a context that could be a high-risk one for such an allegation being believed and acted upon with the professional network rather than being seen as a transference manifestation. The fact that I am a male worker, though he had been abused by his mother and possibly by other adults, also placed me in a vulnerable position in terms of working with sexual abuse, because such abuse is so readily associated with the notion of the male perpetrator. In addition, the fact that I was not seeing him in a clinic setting, with, for instance, colleagues in the next room, served to heighten the issue in terms of containing professional anxiety within the network.

Jim was seen in the same context as the three patients I have described, but with different professional personnel involved, and a great deal of time and effort was spent in endeavouring to ensure that there was a sound working relationship within the professional network. There was, however, something fundamentally different about this experience which, I believe, goes further than that being explicable in terms of these different professional people and which serves to illuminate a part of the child's pathology.

The referral and early therapy

I have not met his mother, but I think that it is of immense importance to understand something of her history and frame of mind in order to understand Jim. Reports describe how she appeared to have been badly abused, physically, emotionally, and sexually, by her own parents. Additionally, she was perceived as being fundamentally disturbed by this abuse and seemed to repeat the damaging behaviour in her adult life. The extent of her disturbance was reflected in her confusion between her dreams, fantasies, and memories. She had apparently spoken to her social worker of having sex in the back of a car with her father, of bad dreams of her brother getting into bed with her, and of masturbating while imagining that her father was doing this. In all these conversations, she was not clear whether they were dreams or actual recollections.

When Jim was referred to therapy he was no longer living with his mother, but there were immense concerns regarding his behaviour. He could be very withdrawn but at other times would explode with immense anger. He could not be trusted to be left alone with animals or younger children and had been found with his finger in the anus of a dog, and he seemed very preoccupied with children's bottoms and vaginas. He had also been known to self-mutilate, severely scratching his own face and groin.

At the start of therapy, it was very difficult to see him alone. He seemed overwhelmed by anxiety at the thought of his foster mother leaving the room. Gradual interpretation of both the separation anxiety and the fear of being alone with me led to independent sessions. In some of these sessions, he would often explore quite sexualized material and seemed to show anxiety that I would want to abuse him or enter some kind of sexualized relationship with him.

Jim did exhibit sexualized behaviour in the room and did at times remove his clothes. Sometimes he also wet his clothes by urinating in them, but also through his play with the water. I kept a spare set of clothes for him. This was all known within the professional framework.

At times his behaviour was also very puzzling and anxiety provoking to me, a fact that had led me to seek consultation on the case with an experienced, senior colleague. The session after which he made his accusation had itself been discussed in depth in consultation; interestingly, the session had been marked by the complete absence of the previous behaviour that had caused so much concern. This was commented on within the consultation prior to my being aware of the allegation.

The arrangement for consultation was made before the session with Jim, and the session was therefore written-up carefully. It was not the sort of session that I might normally have thought of recording in detail or of discussing within the professional network. I hold a model of professional confidentiality where, if there are particular sessions in which a child exhibits behaviour that could easily be subject to misrepresentation, I ensure that this is well recorded and that the general and, if needs be, particular points of concern are known to the appropriate professional colleagues. It is important to distinguish between confidentiality and secrecy, especially as the latter is such an issue for abused children.

I had been meeting with Jim for some nine months prior to the break forced by the allegation. During this time I had built up a good working partnership with the professional network, including the foster parents. This partnership seemed open, and we had discussed the difficulties that they were experiencing, including the foster mother's fears that Jim might make some allegation against her or her partner. The professional network was also aware of the struggle that this presented for me as a therapist working with Jim, but the consensus was that it was important to maintain therapy and to endeavour to work through these issues.

The allegation

I think it might be useful to relate the events as they occurred, as they are illustrative of some of the difficulties that colleagues might experience in similar cases. Jim had returned to therapy after the Easter break. The following week I was informed by the foster mother that he was not well, though I had also been informed that he had begun at a playgroup and it did seem odd that he was well enough to attend that. The next week I was given similar information, and I spoke to the key social worker, saying that I felt that things did not add up and was wondering what was happening. He confirmed that Jim was not well. This continued for three weeks, with my sensing that there was something strange going on but being unable to put my finger on quite what it was. There was then a telephone call from the police saying that they wanted to talk to me. I presumed that this was over another case in which, interestingly, there were strong suggestions of professional abuse by a childcare worker. When I managed to speak to the police officer, he mentioned that he wanted to speak to me regarding Jim but could not at this point divulge why. We arranged a meeting, my presumption now being that perhaps there were further court cases regarding his earlier life history prior to being accepted into care and that the police were wanting an opinion. I was left perplexed as to why the social worker had not spoken to me of this but was unable to get further clarification. When the police officers met with me, they began by endeavouring to make it clear that they were meeting with me to seek information rather than interviewing a suspect for an offence. They then described how Jim had told the social worker that I had interfered with him. I was informed that a case conference had been held and a diagnostic interview. Though I was very shocked, I was also relieved that I could now make sense of my recent experience.

The police seemed very conversant with the issues of child abuse and with the concept of transference and were very sensitive and supportive. Their report said that they felt that there was no substance to the allegations and that Jim should resume therapy as soon as possible. When I contacted the social workers, concerned to clarify matters, I was given the following information. After the session Jim had told his foster mother that I had removed his trousers and played with his penis and that I had also given him some red medication to make him go to sleep. She had then discussed this with the foster agency social worker who had quite rightly taken it up with the social services department (SSD) that referred Jim, with the SSD where he lives, and with the social workers where I live. The network in this case was very complicated and involved a private fostering agency, three SSDs and two police authorities. A decision was made to hold a diagnostic interview, in which Jim firmly repeated the allegations. The team of social workers and police felt that it was a transference issue but decided that the police should complete their own investigations. A number of people had by this time been informed of the allegation and of the measures that were being taken, all, of course, unknown to me. The case conference decision was that Jim was not to return to therapy until the police investigation had been completed. There seemed to be some hiccup in the procedure as it took several weeks for the investigation to be completed. My own opinion is that some time limit should have been placed on procedures at this first meeting and a second case conference held to close the matter. After the police met with me, the SSD did not seem to feel that it was their responsibility to hold a further case conference. I was told by the team manager that they viewed their brief as that of child protection in a limited sense of safety and physical protection and 'moved on to the next case'. It was very much left to me to ensure that my name was cleared and for me and the agency social worker to try to plan for Jim's return to therapy. This seemed to reflect a poor balance between a quite rigid child-protection brief and the more complex issues of the impact of this experience upon the child and upon the credibility of the professional involved.

After an inexplicably long period of time and pressure from me that this matter should be formally closed, the police in the child's area of residence eventually wrote a note saying that I had been interviewed and it was decided that no further action would be taken in respect of the matter. This was clearly an inadequate document in terms of my needs as it placed me in the same category as someone with whom there was strong suspicion but lack of firm evidence. Given that the SSD would not hold a formal case conference, a planning meeting had to be held, attended by my local SSD representative together with the investigating police and the agency social worker. Apologies for non-attendance were sent from the other two SSDs. I had also had a discussion with my professional association, the Association of Child Psychotherapists, which it was very useful to call upon as an external authority. The police officer again made clear his position and was in full agreement that the note written by his colleague in the other police department was inadequate. He allowed his earlier report, which detailed matters more coherently, to be circulated to all parties. It all highlighted the inadequacy of procedures, in that I had to provide the impetus to ensure that all parties who had been told of the alleged abuse were also informed that there was absolutely no substance to the allegations.

Although it had only been my work with Jim that had been interrupted, my local SSD now recommended that I be allowed to continue to meet with children and supervise staff, and I was given clearance that I was not seen to be a danger to my own children! Such is the manner in which such an investigation can invade one's professional and personal life.

Impact upon the therapist

Situations like this place an inevitable strain on all the professionals involved as they erode the very fabric of open, mutually supportive, and trusting professional relationships. They place, however, a particular, if obvious, strain upon the alleged abuser as she or he has to struggle with a very disturbing awareness of being seen in such a light. I certainly found the experience extremely stressful and feel very fortunate in having a very supportive wife and family as well as supportive friends and colleagues. I think that it is vital to acknowledge that, if such an allegation were to be made when the alleged abuser was, for whatever reason, already in a vulnerable state, the consequences could be quite catastrophic. When I was first informed of the allegation, I was left feeling very angry, not so much with Jim but at the way in which the matter was handled. I was also aware of a feeling that might well have arisen however it had been managed: an internal voice of incredulity that my integrity had been in some way doubted. This I had to try simultaneously to reconcile with an awareness of the necessity for correct child protection procedures. I was also very anxious about the other children whom I saw in therapy, and even now, some considerable time after the incident, I feel concerned that if further allegations are made by other children, they will be linked to this incident and I will, as a consequence, be treated with added suspicion. I fear there is no way that one's name can be completely cleared once such an allegation has been made.

That the allegation also led to a statement as regards my relationship to my own children filled me with a deeper despair. This sentence really brought the matter home to me. I then realized with a vengeance that there had been the possibility of further and very distressing consequences to my personal life and that of my family. This could have been completely shattered. I had become increasingly furious at how uncontained things had felt and at how difficult it had proved to ensure that whoever had been told of the allegation was also informed that my name had been cleared. This last statement – 'not a danger to my own children' which meant that prior to that it was considered as a possibility – really underlined the point. I do not think that the serious impact of the allegation of abuse upon myself as the alleged abuser was adequately borne in mind by the child protection officers. This experience really highlighted for me the very real danger that, if such matters are not thoroughly considered and, of utmost importance, 'contained', they become in themselves a form of professional abuse.

Understandably, I felt very cautious about resuming work with Jim. I stood to lose a great deal, and before taking him back into therapy I had to ensure that an appropriate framework existed in case there were any future allegations.

Planning the return to therapy

Through a range of discussions with various colleagues I arrived at the following proposal.

1. If it was possible, as it was important for Jim's development, therapy should be resumed, but there was no reason to presume

that there would not be repeated allegations in the future.

2. Future sessions would be tape-recorded as a way of balancing child protection issues and the need to protect myself. This would, in a way, play into the very pathology that I was trying to work through, but it seemed unavoidable in terms of protecting my professional credibility.

3. Following audio taping, a senior colleague would, if any further allegations were made, be able to listen to the recordings and act as an 'incident assessor' and to avoid a repeat of the break in therapy and the difficult diagnostic procedure that had been experienced –unless this were to prove absolutely necessary.

There are, of course, recognizable shortcomings in using this proposal as a safety net, but I feel that some of these are inevitable as one is seeking a procedural solution to a psychological problem. There was, for instance, some pressure to install video facilities, but what happens with a child who is too young or too frightened to go to the toilet alone? Does one also install a camera in the toilet, or can one only do this work if a colleague is permanently available to cover any eventuality?

Comment

In Freud's paper on 'transference-love' (1915a), he makes the very important distinction between 'acting out' and 'remembering' and sees them as opposite and antithetical paths for bringing the past into the present. 'Acting out' is seen to occur in the motor sphere of action, remembering in the 'psychical sphere' of mentalization and verbalization. 'Acting out' remains faithful to its origins and does not undergo the same transforming process of reconstruction that a memory inevitably does. In discussing 'transference-love', Freud describes how 'if the patient's advances were returned ... she would have succeeded ... in acting out, in repeating in real life, what she ought only to have remembered, to have reproduced as psychical material and to have kept within the sphere of psychical events' (p. 166).

Searle (1969), in the development of 'speech-act' theory, usefully shows how in certain verbal expressions this distinction is not clear. Some statements – such as 'I declare the Olympics open', are performative, and some specific acts can only be performed in words. These are acts in the guise of psychical expressions (Stern, 1993). The expression 'X has alleged that Y abused him' carries with it, in certain circumstances, this sense of action within the words and, as such, is a statement that can of itself lead to a radical, and irretrievable, change in a relationship.

With Jim, the decision to hold a case conference and to stop therapy blurred the distinction between 'acting out' and 'remembering'. The experience of an allegation being made, and acted upon, then placed the key figures in the system, child, therapist, social worker, foster parent, and so on, in a very different state from what they were in before. It was important not only to recognize the conscious difficulties that might arise from this, but also to pay due attention to the unconscious processes that might influence and subvert the way in which the situation was managed. In these circumstances the key figures become organized in a way more akin to what Bentovim (1992) describes as a 'trauma-organized system', and, if resources are available, it would be useful to engage an external consultant formally at this point. The impact on the child, the therapist, and the relationship between them is likely to be extreme, as, too, is that between the therapist and the professional network. The social worker and foster mother had, for example, been forced to entertain the idea that I, as a colleague whom they trusted and to whom they had sent a child in their care, might also be an abuser. In consequence, they had both felt obliged to lie to me. I, for my part, had to struggle with being seen in this light and being lied to.

Working with any child that has been multiply abused places immense strain upon the therapist and the professional network. There is a constant pressure to enact with the patient his or her perverse internal object relationships. In this case, thinking about the networks as a whole, the correct decision to hold a diagnostic interview meant that the team moved from the 'psychical sphere' and treated this as an experience that might have happened. This has very important repercussions in terms of the child's therapy and whether or not it can be resumed, as it raises the related questions as to whether the relationships between the child and the therapist and between the therapist and the professional network have been irretrievably changed, and, if so, whether they have changed in a way that makes it impossible to continue therapy.

As a team, and after considerable discussions, we decided to continue Jim's therapy. Obviously, the experience was felt to have had an impact upon the relationship between Jim and me, and between the network and me, but this was not felt to be irretrievable. I looked forward – with interest but also undoubted apprehension, to resuming therapy with Jim and to exploring this dynamic in the consulting room.

Jane Milton (1994) describes how hard it is to strike the right balance when working with victims of abuse:

> Sympathetic attention to the person who has been a helpless victim is essential. At the same time it is vital to address what is perhaps the most serious aspect of the victim's plight: her corruption in childhood via excessive stimulation of her own hatred and destructiveness, which becomes eroticized, and her identification with the aggressor, often as a means of psychic survival (Milton, 1994, p. 243)

Jim had been badly abused as a child, and it was, of course, important to pay sympathetic attention to this; at the same time it was vital to keep in mind the corruption that had occurred in his childhood and the possible identification with the aggressor. Much of my apprehension as regards resuming therapy with Jim rested upon my experience as a 'helpless victim' within a situation brought about through his actions.

Return to therapy

We had decided that it would be best to have a meeting between the social worker, the foster mother, Jim, and me in order to go through what had happened and to offer Jim some explanation as regards continuing therapy and the safeguards that we had decided to implement, most importantly, the use of a tape recorder in the sessions. At this session, Jim arrived 'full of beans', quickly settling to his toys and behaving in a quite jovial way. He played separately from the adult group, and we, as a group, felt it important for him to come over and to listen to what was being discussed. The events were run over, and Jim was asked to contribute to this. The whole tone of the session then became quite different and very sober. Jim was silent when asked to recount the events, and his foster mother struggled to encourage him to relate what had happened and what he had told her. This part of the session felt very uncomfortable and persecutory, but, as Jim and his foster mother related the events, I could quite see how the allegation was taken seriously. Importantly, in terms of the countertransference this whole procedure felt quite unreal, as I struggled to listen to what was being related and process this alongside my own memory of the session.

The social worker explained how important returning to therapy was and that the sessions would be recorded so that, in the future, if Jim felt after a session that I had done something, he could again tell his foster mother and the tape could then be listened to, to see if he had confused his memory of the sessions and what actually happened. This would protect him and me from further police investigations, unless they were felt to be absolutely necessary.

This part of the session was then drawn to a close, and the social worker and the foster mother left. The tone of things had gradually grown more light-hearted, and Jim spoke of feeling OK at being left alone with me.

This encounter was obviously very different from the normal events of long-term work with a child. I felt that procedurally it was necessary if therapy was to continue, but it felt bizarre and confusing. It was important to bear in mind during the meeting that Jim had been through a number of investigative interviews, the impact of which would have been different from those of the primary trauma. The role of the investigator, establishing what had happened, was clearly different from that of the therapist, and the role of the child in a diagnostic interview was likewise different. This meeting was attempting to bridge that gap.

I was certainly working in an atmosphere beyond my experience as a child psychotherapist, but the disassociation that I experienced between my memory of the session and how it was being recounted by Jim, and the split between his light-hearted/jovial and sombre/persecuted state, also reminded me that in cases of childhood sexual abuse the victim can enter into a disassociated state as a result of the trauma (Putnam, 1985).

The whole issue of the use of the tape recorder also meant that there was still a certain amount of necessary 'acting out' going on, in the sense of the continuing need for a physical as opposed to a psychological reaction to the events.

The role of the tape recorder

For a number of months after the return to therapy, this split between a rather light-hearted/jovial and sombre/persecuted mode of relating was in evidence in most sessions. The tape recorder played a key role in this. Jim would often begin the sessions in a jovial mood where the whole affect was quite light-hearted, but quite often, for reasons that I could not always ascertain, the tone of the sessions would change. He seemed to become frightened, and either before or after this change in mood he would ask again and again what the recorder was for. I have not used a recorder before, and obviously in these sessions it had a special significance. At the beginning of his return to therapy, I was interested to see how things would develop. What seemed to emerge was that, far from the recorder being thought of as neutral or unobtrusive, its presence had to be engaged with actively. My response to his questions was factual and interpretive, focusing on the use of the tape recorder to validate what really happened and how difficult it might sometimes be to differentiate between what happened and what he thought might have happened. After several months, he said to me, 'You didn't really do anything to me did you?' and this led to a fruitful and serious discussion of the course of events and just how confused he sometimes became as regards his memory of events. His supposition when in the accusatory frame of mind that I had sent him to sleep through the use of a drug obviously added to the confusion and the difficulty of differentiating fantasy from reality. It is also important to note that drugs were thought to be part of the original abusive experience.

Discussion

I felt that Jim's confusion was genuine and, to use a very apposite expression, that he had been an 'honest liar'. In a way that has obvious parallels to the description of his own mother's state of mind, I think that, when he made the allegation, Jim himself genuinely believed in what he was saying. It is, I believe, this quality that crucially differentiates this patient from the first three described above and it is the same quality that led to the allegation being acted upon.

In furthering my understanding of this, I found Michael Sinason's (1993) concept of internal cohabitation or co-residency of two minds in one body very useful as a working model. He starts from Freud's concept of the way in which, if an ego is overwhelmed by demands of the external worlds, a process of detachment can take place whereby part of the ego then remains orientated by the demands of the external reality while the detached part lives in the world of illusions (Freud, 1924e). Rosenfeld's

(1971) elaboration of this:

> illustrated how an internal psychic organization can be built up within the ego and turns them to destructive ends. Intelligence is thereby turned to the service of destructiveness; and achievement is conceived of solely in terms of the domination and subjugation of others to the narcissistic aims of the ill ego. (M. Sinason, 1993, p. 209; cf. Patient B above).

Rosenfeld develops the notion of the internal gang, whereby treatment is then conceived of as disentangling the residual sane parts of the ego from the destructive narcissistic parts. Sinason expands this concept, describing how he conceives of treatment as fostering the development in the patient of a genuine capability for making decisions in life which adequately take account of the needs of his own mind as well as that of the cohabitee. He describes how treatment

> cannot be achieved by premature injunctions for the patient to 'be responsible' and will not occur if the patient has an attitude of wishing to be rid of the co-habitee or of condemnation and resentment. One important part of the development of genuine interest and concern for the co-habitee comes through attention to the ways in which the mind of the co-habitee is often using concrete symbolic equations instead of symbolism and is therefore unable to think symbolically, which constitutes a significant degree of thought disorder and disability. This in turn leads to a recognition that destructive consequences do not always rise from destructive aims. A mind that is incapable of symbolic functioning can be urgent, ruthless and expedient and thereby injure others directly as a result of these disabilities. (M. Sinason, 1993, p. 219)

The links with the differentiation between 'acting out' and 'remembering' will be apparent, as will the difficulties of the professional network in moving from the psychical to the physical domain, for at that point the network can be said to have been in the service of this disabled part of the mind.

Further clinical material illustrates this more clearly. Jim would often play at the sink. He would almost always ask me to come close when engaged in this activity, and, though I would explore this with him, it was not possible to fully ascertain the reasons for this. The split between light-hearted/jovial and sombre/persecuting was again apparent in his play. He would often seem happily engaged but then suddenly become frightened. In one session, he leapt back in real terror, eventually being able to say that he was frightened of 'the monster in the sink … look, there are its eyes'. He was pointing to the plug, and, as the last drops of water went down the pipe, I could imagine how they could be seen as eyes. The 'trigger' for his anxiety and his reaction was unusually in the open, and we could discuss his confusion. He then put a flannel over the plug. It helped momentarily, but he then said, 'But it's still in there, only covered up'.

This provides an illustration of Jim's mental processes and, at this point in time, the lack of symbolic functioning. There are obvious parallels between this and the allegation of abuse and, perhaps most poignantly with reference to the tape recorder, his fear that the abuser was still lurking within me. There are also important differences, the most pertinent of which is that with this material I was able to take it up psychically and think it through with him.

Looking for triggers

What, though, of the specific aetiology of the allegation of abuse? Why did this particular child respond in this way? I think further clues to understanding this can be found in the experience of holiday breaks and the primitive, infantile feelings that may be aroused at those times. In order to understand the material, it was important to think about the ways in which Jim's earliest and most primitive interactions with his primary objects would have left their traces, exerting a powerful but disabling and destructive influence upon the form and structure of his personality.

The first holiday break after his return was dominated by a planned change of foster parents. Following the next break (Easter and the anniversary of the time at which he had alleged the abuse), Jim did not return for his first session and I was left waiting for him, very anxiously! I later telephoned the foster home and was informed that the session had been forgotten! At the next session, when Jim did return he was physically sick on the way. This had not happened at any other time, and I believe that this and the previously forgotten session were more than coincidence and had to do with the anniversary of the allegation. In the following session with Jim, I made an interpretation along these lines, and he nodded in agreement.

Some months later, at the last session before the summer break, the recorder again became the focus of his attention. Jim had become quite aggressive, and I had been interpreting this material with regards to the impending summer break when he responded by saying that I could turn the recorder off. This, I think, provides a vital clue, as it demonstrates how in his mind he links the experience of my 'turning the sessions off' with that of being able to turn the recorder off and, presumably, in his phantasy, then taking away the recorder's protective capacity and leaving him open to further abuse.

Freud presumed childhood love to be boundless: 'It demands exclusive possession. It is not content with less than all. But it has a second characteristic: it has in point of fact no aim and is incapable of obtaining complete satisfaction; and principally for this reason it is doomed to end in disappointment and to give place to a hostile attitude.'

The material that Jim presented in the sessions does then lend itself to linking the allegation of abuse to these hostile, early infantile feelings, reactivated in therapy at the holiday breaks but jaundiced by his real-life experiences of gross sexual abuse and a problematic infancy with a mother with severe mental health problems. He has a long, repetitive history of changing primary carers; the break from his mother was because of concerns as regards her capacity to look after her children and allegations of sexual abuse. His history links separations to allegations of sexual abuse and this seemed to be the destructive quality that was acted upon at the point at which the allegation was made.

Conclusion

In this chapter I have focused on a specific situation, a false allegation of sexual abuse, in which a patient's communications and memories of a particular event seemed to transform that event radically and with potentially drastic results. Through an exploration of work with a number of other patients, who for varying reasons have made varying allegations of abuse against myself as their therapist, I have tried to consider and differentiate between different frames of mind and, especially, to explore some of the reasons behind this particular allegation being believed and acted upon in contrast to others that were not. The very fact that the allegation was believed did seem to throw some light upon the patient's own pathology and his own belief, at that point, that something had really happened. This belief had a very real impact upon the professional network, resulting in a full diagnostic enquiry and, because professional abuse does take place, this could be considered as necessary 'acting out'. But such 'acting out' can reinforce the disturbed part of the patient's personality and is a most disturbing experience for the therapist, the patient, and other members of the professional network.

CHAPTER 8

Then and now – a historical perspective

Emerald Davis in an interview with Valerie Sinason

Emerald is an Afro-Caribbean woman born in Guyana, who came to the UK at the age of 19. She trained as a nurse, specialized as a psychiatric nurse, a midwife and finally a sister. She then found her lasting home in psychotherapy, training and practising as an attachment-based psychoanalytic psychotherapist with a special interest in disability, dissociation and minorities.

Emerald was vice chair and then chair of the Bowlby Centre for twelve years, until her retirement. She also chaired the Bowlby Centre Ethics Committee for many years, until that function was centralized and transferred to the UK Council for Psychotherapy (UKCP). Under her leadership, great care was taken to ensure the independence of the committee, making the complaints process accessible, thoughtful and supportive to all sides. At present, she maintains a small private practice in South London and continues to offer supervision.

I am grateful for her willingness to be interviewed to contribute to this book.

As a black woman coming to the UK in your teens would you consider a lot of your early experiences should and could have been subject for a complaint?

Yes. I arrived in the UK at the age of 19 under the auspices of the British Council to embark on psychiatric nurse training. I was shocked to realize that in my first three months I was only allowed to work as a domestic. When I approached the Matron she flatly informed me that she could not consider me for the training until I learned English and I had to complete an English Course (even though that was my actual language!).

Well it took me another few months and with the subtle help of an Irish Staff Nurse, I managed to get myself out of that situation and into another psychiatric training hospital to do my training. After successfully completing the training, I applied to another hospital to do my SRN (State Registered Nurse) training and again met with difficulties. I was initially accepted and then had the agreement rescinded because apparently I was not considerate enough to give back some extra time to my training hospital before moving on. I'm afraid I did not agree with the way I was treated by both hospitals and did not alter my resignation.

I went down to see my cousin in South London and she suggested I stay with her whilst looking for another hospital to continue with my plans for further training. This did not last long as I tried to sign on as unemployed. I think the clerk I spoke with seemed sympathetic and gave me details for another training hospital in South East London. This proved very beneficial to me as I was invited to come in for an interview which was successful and I enjoyed the training and was able to then move on to do my midwifery training.

If something like that happened now it would be upheld as a major complaint so there has been some social improvement. What happened next?

I worked as a midwife for two years and thoroughly enjoyed the work even though I experienced an awful amount of structural and institutional racism. It was always upsetting but I had learnt to deal with most of it. Patients telling me not to touch them with my black hands was awful, but the slurs that came from other members of staff was intolerable. This was not a period where complaints about such treatment would have been accepted.

And then what happened?

I worked in the NHS for some 30 odd years in different disciplines including district nursing and then moved on to working in a GP Practice as a Health Prevention Sister before embarking on a counselling course which led me on to an attachment psychotherapy course.

Did the therapeutic environment feel less racist?

It felt that at last I had found my niche. However, in my first year as a trainee during a group session the facilitator said to me that she didn't know why I was put in her group since she did not know anything about black people. Neither myself or any of my colleagues commented on it. Thinking about it now, she did cross the line and if that were to happen today I would hope that I and other members in the group would have objected as a blatant racial slur. However, what can be reflected on or complained about changes over time.

How did your training affect you?

Because of my own experiences of displacement and not feeling wanted, I was absolutely delighted to find an organization that was in its embryonic stage of development and was open to new ideas. I think I was among the second set of trainees.

These were exciting times for me and I was even able most of the time to put my imposter syndrome aside as I was keen to join in and found myself contributing at every opportunity. The organization's main concept was first formulated by John Bowlby's notion of a secure base – a new approach in working with mental distress. Bowlby was the first in his field to highlight the fact of human beings' need for others. Our core structure of the organization was founded on our vision, mission and values with a focus for attachment-based psychotherapy, with an emphasis on research and community-based development. Also there was a focus for information and training for psychotherapists and health professionals.

Historically, psychoanalytical and psychotherapy had only been available to people who were psychologically minded (the worried well so to speak) and well able to respond and pay for treatment. Clients with psychiatric diagnoses were deemed unsuitable for treatment, as were those from black and minority ethnic communities. These were said to be unable to reflect because of their inferior brains. So race issues were always there for me but the BC (Bowlby Centre) cared about inclusion and gave me a home.

As the training progressed and I became a psychotherapist in training and started to see clients under supervision, I was passionately aware of what a privilege it was to have clients entrust their very vulnerable selves to us in treatment. I was often so grateful for the unshakeable ground rules we had devised and how our values and missions statement cemented the work in our treatment room. Unlike now, these were the early days in first thinking and caring about racially motivated bias and the like. It was exciting to be at the start of such thinking.

How did these experiences inform your later practice?

When I became Chair of the Bowlby Centre I wished for it to be a place that welcomed diversity and reflected on complexity. As it focused on patients who had experienced trauma, as well as providing training for therapists from diverse experiences, I wanted it to be a place where boundary issues and misattunements could be considered reflectively. It was also a relatively small place and people's therapists and supervisors might also be getting therapy within the same group so extra care had to be taken how to balance transparency with confidentiality. I also wanted the environment to be un-shaming.

We understood from the start that our organization wished to contain and aid its members (staff and students) and its patients and that this would be complex for such a small group. It was a relief when we were able to join our organization to the UKCP and pass on complaints to them. However, before this was possible I was determined, for example, that the Ethics Committee should be as independent as possible and that complaints should go to them in the first instance with the concept that mediation should be the first step. We understood that where something was not criminal it was attachment-linked and needed handling with great care, especially as patients/clients seen at the centre were survivors of trauma and we were dealing with problematic issues coming out of therapy.

What were the key issues that became subjects of complaints?

Those with Dissociative Identity Disorder (DID), before the condition was recognized more widely, led to most complaints. A regular composite example would be a situation where a sad and frightened child personality would be given all kinds of extra support beyond the frame in a way that felt over-identified and where a hostile alter-personality attacked this by making a complaint about boundary breaking. These were early days in understanding DID. Extra supervision was provided to look holistically at how treatment of one state could affect the others.

A further composite example would be the situation where the distress of the child state could lead to physical contact, like a hug, which could then cause a switch to an angry adult who saw all touch as abuse. Careful reflection was required here as well as mediation. Sometimes, the patient would continue with the therapist after mediation and sometimes it totally disrupted the attachment. The Ethics Committee would consider whether the practitioner in each case had reflected adequately and, if not, what would enable their learning.

We had to consider: how do you determine where boundary crossing was to enable trust and attachment and where it came from over-identification? How much was it a clinical error to not know a hostile personality might complain? How much clinically should the complaint by one alter be listened to versus the democratic view of all the others?

Ethically, my view would be help for the therapist to understand the impact on other states of what was offered to some as well as appreciating the difficulty. With regard to complaints coming about teachers from students, we had to make sure that our values around respecting diversity were maintained and thought about throughout the training.

What kind of examples came from trainees?

Several were to do with racism. Well here are some amalgamations to illustrate the kind of points. A trainee came out of a seminar and made a throwaway remark about reading a paper written by a 'chinky' to a colleague who was Chinese. This trainee brought the matter to her personal tutor who arranged a meeting between herself, the trainee who made the comment and a member from the Clinical Training Committee (CTC). In the course of the meeting it became clear to the course tutor and the member from the CTC that the trainee was unable to reflect on either her feelings towards her colleague or the reasons for her racist remark. A period for reflection was put aside for the trainee to think about how it felt to be on the receiving end of such a remark and for the course tutor and the member of the CTC to think of a way forward. The trainee however decided to leave the training altogether as she didn't feel ready to own or address her own part in the upsetting exchange.

I've thought a lot about this kind of example because we were so sorry to lose a student and the only way I could logically make sense for myself was that at the BC we prided ourselves on making everyone feel welcome and accepted, warts and all. So when we do say 'no' it can be felt like a punishment and, as it is almost unheard of, it is difficult to accept that some attitudes are not accepted at our organization. I think she felt criticized and maybe shamed? And although that's the last thing we would want, we have to uphold our values. Even though there are subtle and institutional racist throwaway attitudes in the wider communities, we cannot accept it here at the BC.

We offered mediation in an attempt to help her to feel supported but it seemed as though she could only see it as a rejection so it probably felt easier for her to leave.

A student made a complaint because she felt she was unfairly treated and felt the decision was racially biased. She was told that she was not ready as she did not achieve the level of competence expected and needed to write a paper demonstrating that she understood the context/complexities/professional development and that she should also increase her personal therapy sessions. She approached me for advice, support and solidarity. After some discussion, she agreed to write the paper and I was so proud of her as she wrote a brilliant account of where she was at. I was happy to be able to support her in this way but to this day when I reflect on it, I can't help feeling some unease at the way she was treated and I was glad that I was there to give her that much-needed support. Not all results feel right.

A white trainee expressed a difficulty with a black course tutor who brought the issue to the CTC. After some discussion, it was agreed that the trainee be asked to write a reflective paper on her own experience of being discriminated against and how discrimination impacts on the experience of others. She wrote a very thoughtful and detailed piece and felt that she had learned a great deal from the experience. Her supervisor was advised of the issue and provided evidence in her supervisor's report that the trainee was developing a sensitive way of working with difference.

Another trainee expressed a strong aversion to the idea of two women bringing up a child in a lesbian relationship and refused to carry out an infant observation unless the parents were a man and a woman. The trainer brought the matter to the course tutor who raised it with the CTC. The committee decided in the end not to insist on the trainee carrying out the lesbian infant observation but asked the trainee to write a reflective piece on sexuality. The committee also informed the trainee that she would be only be considered for the next term if there was evidence of ongoing thoughtfulness and change. The committee asked all the other trainers to assess very closely and to give feedback on a regular basis, which was done. All four trainers reported an increase in her reflective thinking as a result. Again, this was before the current awareness of LGBT (Lesbian, Gay, Bisexual and Transgender) issues and was pioneering.

The Bowlby Centre is unusual in stating it wishes to support its therapists, patients and the public

The values of the BC were so important that there was a strong wish to do right by patients, therapists, lecturers, staff and students, whether they were making a complaint or receiving one. That was why the good relationship and transparency between the Chair and the Head of Ethics was so important to me. I was very lucky to have someone like Pat Cohen in that role as someone from a diverse background. Because of her own lived experiences and mine of difference it was a good match. As a result of our thinking, we ensured the Ethics Committee could be separate and independent and all complaints could go to it first and then an attempt at mediation if that was felt possible. Mediation was the first hope. And it was to be the first step.

As a training organization were there other areas of complaint that needed thinking about?

Where is the line between good and bad practice? In the grey area of a staff member having a relationship with a student/supervisee, I was aware of building up understanding of where I felt a complaint was justified. Where I felt someone used their power to achieve such a relationship and was unaware of any damage they had caused, I considered they could be dangerous as a therapist. Whereas, although unhelpful, some such relationships were not activated from an abuse of power, I can recall personal upset at a complaint being upheld which I considered harsh as well as situations where someone was able to walk away without consequences, wrongly.

We also had a staff member who after, a complaint, left and joined another organization and that still rests with me: could we have done better?

Final thoughts on complaints?

All my work has been attachment-based whether as a therapist, a lecturer or as Chair of an organization. I think values are extremely important and helping people in an inclusive, un-shaming way to understand what has happened, what had gone wrong, to offer mediation. But even that cannot always create a happy ending for the complained about or complainant.

PART III

TOWARDS THE FUTURE

CHAPTER 9

The unique nature of boundaries in psychoanalytic therapy and the implication for ethics and complaints procedures

Philip Stokoe

Introductory remarks

The work of the psychoanalytic psychotherapist creates a unique challenge to the design of ethical codes, complaints and disciplinaries. This is because the work occurs at the boundary. The fact that we work on the boundary and will frequently be drawn across it means that our registering bodies should design ethical codes that reflect that reality. The unprofessional conduct cannot be defined as crossing a boundary but remaining there (Stokoe, 2020, p. 122), and the unconscious to unconscious pressures cannot be exaggerated.

The location of psychoanalytic work is a relationship but not a 'normal' relationship. It is based on the psychoanalytic assumption that our problems, by which I mean our emotional and psychological problems, originate in beliefs, habits of mind or assumptions about ourselves and the world we live in that are held 'unconsciously'. That means that we are not directly aware of these ideas, only of the implications deriving from them in the way we see the world around us. Therapeutic work involves an emotional engagement that allows exploration of the patient's mind by the therapist. This means that a normal boundary between two people has to become permeable. The consequence is that the ethical codes and the complaints procedures have to be designed around *dynamic* rather than static boundaries.

The implications for successful help are:

- that the individual comes to the view that they need help, that is, that they have a problem
- the person providing the help is able to perceive the unconscious blockages to healthy function, and
- that they can activate and recruit the curiosity of the individual requiring help in areas that have previously been taken to be absolute, concrete facts.

I want to consider briefly the means to discovering someone else's unconscious functioning and the ways in which we might reactivate someone's curiosity, because both of these processes have implications for the formality of the setting in which helpers work. My thesis in this chapter is that those implications make psychotherapy very different from other professions.

You never told me you were going to …

Many psychoanalysts have written about the situation in which the analyst or therapist behaves in an unprofessional way (Gabbard, 1995, 2000). These studies are very helpful in anticipating the personality problems that might lead a clinician to lose contact with their professional task and enter a different type of relationship. My own experience of this area started shortly after I had qualified as an organizational consultant at the Tavistock Clinic in London in 1983. I was invited to advise on how to deal with the disciplinary process involving a deputy manager of a residential social work unit who was accused of stealing petty cash. I found myself wondering how many residential social workers were disciplined compared to field social workers. I should say that I had been a manager of a therapeutic unit in a specialist, secure centre for adolescents and had acquired considerable experience of the unconscious pressures on staff in such environments. The reader may not be surprised to learn that 90 per cent of disciplinaries within social service departments were against residential social workers. The management who dealt with such disciplinaries must have been aware of this, but their lack of enquiry into it suggested that they hadn't really noticed or had not seen it as significant. I wondered, why? This led me to think about the period leading up to the event that triggered the enquiry. Was there a process that made sense of the behaviour? For instance, was it that this person was essentially untrustworthy and had chosen residential work because it was an ideal environment to act out? Alternatively, was there something going on in the complex intercourse between clients and social workers that might have had such a strong impact on this individual that they found themselves taking small amounts of cash designed for the everyday needs of those clients? My research into this case led to just such a story: a story so clear that it led the disciplinary panel not only to acquit the individual but, at my suggestion, to instigate weekly support meetings for the staff team to help them discover the impacts that the unconscious exchanges between their clients and themselves were having on each of them.

This led me to formulate a principle which I have applied to all of my work with supervisees, professional clients, organizations and teams since. I always start from the assumption that they are committed professionals trying to do a good job and that any behaviour or comments that seem to suggest otherwise must be unconscious expressions of the emotional material emanating from the work. This means that my first task is to search for whatever in the work might account for this behaviour. Usually something does, and that allows us to understand it so that it ceases to hold the individual in its grip. Sometimes no such explanation occurs, in which case we have proved that this issue really does belong to the personality of the individual. I shall expand on this later, but it represents my experience that the unconscious-to-unconscious-pressures cannot be exaggerated.

> 'It is a very remarkable thing that the Ucs. of one human being can react upon that of another, without passing through the Cs.'
> (Freud, 1915e, p. 194)

As well as that working principle, I learnt that the claim against the member of staff, whatever the specific wording, was always an expression of the formula, 'you never told me you were going to …'. The dots can be filled in with examples such as, 'steal from me', 'exploit me', 'threaten me' or 'have sex with me'. In other words, the complaint raised in my mind the question, 'So, what did the professional say *would* happen?'

Putting it another way, any investigation of a complaint has to begin at the start of the professional relationship if there is any chance to make sense of it. Starting at the point of the complaint is bound to lose the narrative that will make sense of what is now complained about. Sadly, most psychoanalytic studies of complaints begin with the complaint itself. In my view, the complaint is the *end* of a process and you can only understand it properly by looking at what led up to that point.

I have indicated that the therapeutic work involves an unconscious impact on the clinician and that this can have a massive effect. The most common means by which this occurs is through projective identification and, although we can be aware that something has been stirred up within us, because we cannot see our own unconscious, we might well attribute it to something about us and, therefore, miss the discovery that it is actually something about our patient. The ubiquity of this phenomenon is why psychotherapy institutions insist that their members receive supervision. It is why I had recommended to that social service department that their residential staff receive staff support meetings. The reason is simple. We might not notice these unconscious impacts on us, but it is extremely likely that our colleagues will. In other words, the same principle that says that the unconscious determinants of a patient's problem will only be visible to someone else, applies to clinicians too.

Since the first ideas about psychoanalytic therapy were presented, the characteristics of the venue of the work became an important area for agreement. Over time, this has come to be described as the 'setting' or the 'frame'. The design of the setting was based on the understanding that the main material for analysis would be the way that the patient related to the analyst. The assumption was that those beliefs that distort a patient's view of himself in relation to others or to the world would be revealed in his relationship to the analyst. In order to *maximize* this phenomenon, it would be essential to *minimize* the true nature of the analyst's personality or life circumstances. The physical setting should be as impersonal as possible, and the analyst should retain an evenly suspended attention (Freud 1912e and 1923a). This is what I would like to call the therapeutic container.

The therapeutic and the secondary containers

If the work happens at the boundary and if this is a sort of emotional struggle in which the therapeutic relationship is the site of the struggle, then there must be times when the therapeutic container will crack.

My first encounter with boundaries followed my promotion to manager of a therapeutic unit of a secure provision for dangerous adolescents.

> One of my earliest duties was to decide at what age we'd allow them to smoke (these were the days when everyone smoked). I found it an extremely difficult decision to make, continually unable to balance all the factors ... After several days of indecision, I managed to extricate myself from the morass of pros and cons and look again at the task. It dawned on me that I was overwhelmed with the consequence of a belief that I was supposed to make the 'right' decision...
>
> ... My conscious attempt to find the 'correct' rule was based on a less conscious idea that the correctness of the rule would be accepted by all parties and, therefore, not a source of conflict or complaint. (Stokoe, 2020, pp. 110–111)

Further thinking led me to the realization that a good boundary in the context of the therapeutic task was one that offered an opportunity exactly for what I had unconsciously been trying to avoid, namely a lively encounter between staff and patients. In fact, part of the work of designing a 'safe container' was to recognize that violence was almost always the result of a patient's frustration not being picked up early enough; sensitive, thoughtfully designed rules enabled both staff and adolescents to pick up the tension long before it escalated into violence.

The next observation was that real (therapeutic) work always and only occurred at a boundary. Although useful development of skills and confidence would take place when the adolescents were using the environment appropriately, this was something that followed a usually painful or challenging discovery about their unconscious mind. Those discoveries *always* involved a boundary challenge: for instance, the perception of a member of staff as someone they really were not, through transference or projective identification. This would become manifest in the way the young person treated them disrespectfully or inappropriately – a boundary violation. We had developed the skills to recognize these events as opportunities to explore the unconscious meaning for that young person.

Part of the setting is the definition of the weirdness of the relationship we offer our patients, namely, 'you are a patient and can say or do whatever you like without censorship'; 'I am the therapist and shall attempt to understand the unconscious meaning of whatever you say or do'. As soon as we recognize that these statements are boundaries, then we can see that, for the patient to treat us as an angry father, is to violate the boundary (we are therapists, not angry fathers, we leave that outside the room). It is this assault on the boundary that should trigger the therapist to act. The action, when it is consistent with his part of the therapeutic agreement, will be to interpret the patient's need to 'assault' him in this way. He might link something that has just happened in the room to a belief that the patient holds about his own father.

We do not always notice what the patient has done to us. Sometimes it is only when we notice that we are behaving somewhat tetchily or feeling cross with the patient that we realize what is happening. Sometimes it is only after we have fallen into an argument, that we realize what is going on here. The point is that we often only know that we are picking up something from the patient's unconscious because we notice that we have crossed a boundary (Brenman Pick, 1985; Casement, 1985; Carpy, 1989).

At these times, the saving quality is the arousal of curiosity. The skilled therapist uses his interpretation to arouse the interest/curiosity of the patient, but it is also the curiosity of the therapist that finally causes him to think about what is happening to *him*. The earliest references to the K-drive were about something Freud and Klein thought of as the epistemophilic instinct. For them, this was not an innate drive but a fascination with sex or a fascination with mother's body. The point was that it always involved a wish to break through a personal boundary, either into the parental bedroom or into the body of the parent. Enquiries always have this sense of 'uncovering' something. Our work is about uncovering the truth, so we will inevitably open boundaries. This is how I have previously described the way psychoanalysis should think about rules or boundaries:

They are not 'things' that exist independently of the activities of the working couple, they are part of the engagement of that couple. In fact, they act to stimulate conflict. Perhaps it is truer to say that they are not concrete 'rules' that prescribe the behaviour of the participants, as in a legal contract; they are emotional and psychological material that can be stretched and distorted so as to reveal unconscious information. The skill of the therapist and the therapeutic institution is to maintain a psychological balance that allows these apparent rules to be broken without ever completely losing the Hippocratic commitment to do no harm. (Stokoe, 2020, p. 110)

Nevertheless, it must be apparent that, if the work is constantly on the boundary, this places a massive strain there. I prefer to call the place in which all of this work takes place a 'therapeutic container' and I do so to invoke Bion's concept of container/contained. This is a dynamic concept, not only a relationship between the container and the contained (usual mother and baby) but also an internal relationship between the container and an inner containing object. Indeed, without this, the mother's capacity to provide a sense of containment to the baby will be seriously compromised. You could say that the internal arrangement represents the mother's capacity to move to a third position from which to observe her encounter with her baby. This is similar to the idea of the internal supervisor providing support in an identical configuration to the therapist in relationship with his patient. In the same way that a mother requires someone else to take over when things become a strain, so there will be times when the impact on the therapeutic container makes it crack and break.

If we anticipate that these things are bound to happen from time to time, it is not only reasonable but actually a *duty* to provide for such a circumstance. I propose the concept of secondary container to meet this need. The secondary container is the place where both parties can go to get help when things seem to have broken down. It is also an *actual* 'third position' that can enable the therapist to get help to think about what is happening in his relationship with his patient. The secondary container, therefore, includes the provision of supervision and clinical discussion with fellow professionals. In my experience as a senior manager in the NHS and other health and social care providers, the secondary container is also the place that receives complaints. I have been lucky enough to have been able to ensure that the approach I am describing here could be put into effect in those places.

The first thing to say about the secondary container is that its purpose is to contain and protect the work. It is easy to see how this is done in supervision and clinical discussion, but I should say something about the way it appears when the therapeutic container has broken. At this point, the secondary container acts to provide a place where both patient and therapist are able to think what has gone wrong. This is usually the result of a complaint by the patient (or third party) or the result of anxiety on the part of a supervisor or clinical colleagues. Wherever the concern originates, the action should be to enable the therapist to stop being a therapist and become an equal party to understanding what seems to have gone wrong. I should point out that this does not necessarily mean a meeting between patient, therapist and a representative of the secondary container; if the complaint or anxiety has come from a colleague or supervisor, the discussion might be limited to the therapist and a manager. If the complaint has come from the patient, initial discussions should be between management and patient and, separately, between management and therapist. It may appear to all parties that a three-way meeting would be helpful, but this should not be a default assumption. The reason for this is that what is taking place is a benign enquiry into what appears to have gone wrong. The aim for this enquiry is to see whether the patient's therapy can be protected. The primary aim is to protect the work, not to seek to blame either party. To this end, the enquiry should begin with the start of therapy, not the point at which the therapeutic container broke down. This enables a proper understanding of the process that led to that event. Only an understanding of such a process will provide a full perspective on the event of the breakdown. Once that is understood, the secondary container can suggest actions to be taken both to protect the therapy and to manage concerns about either party.

It has been my experience that this kind of facility in a therapeutic institution produces an agreed way forward in over 90 per cent of cases. Please note that I am not suggesting that protecting the patient's therapy means forcing them to stay with a therapist with whom they cannot work. Quite the opposite; it makes it possible to be clear exactly why another therapist is a sensible move. Very occasionally the outcome is that therapy should not continue at all because it is not appropriate.

I have described the secondary container that can be created within a therapeutic institution. There is no reason why this kind of provision should not or cannot be provided by the registering or membership body to which the therapist belongs. In fact, I think that it is the duty of these bodies to provide exactly this service. Sadly, those in the United Kingdom have decided against such a provision and have chosen to ignore the special nature of boundaries in psychoanalytic work and, instead, have modelled their complaints and ethics systems on those professions in which boundaries can properly be described in black-and-white terms. In simple terms, this has changed a membership body from a place that could provide respectful containment for both patient and therapist, into one that treats its own member as a potential criminal. This has resulted in unnecessary complexity in the process of hearing a complaint; a complexity that begins with the imitation of a court deciding whether a complaint, on the balance of probabilities, has merit and should proceed to a formal enquiry. Neither patient nor therapist feels contained in this process, the one having become the accused and the other the accuser.

The reader might imagine, therefore, the difficulty that those of us who act as expert witnesses in such cases face. Our role is to introduce to people who think they are part of a judicial panel, the concepts of therapeutic complexity, on the one hand, and compassion for both parties on the other. It is a sad irony that I am describing a process of restoring an idea that you only get close to the truth about something if you can take account of the unconscious process underlying the apparent behaviour – this idea having been given up in favour of a superficial, cognitive-level assessment of guilt or innocence.

The complaint

I have said that a complaint, 'you never told me you were going to...' is often perceived in a very concrete way as 'you breached a boundary'. This enables the investigator to fall into the error of believing that the job is to ascertain whether or not such a violation of a boundary occurred. This simplistic approach is based on a premise that a boundary is a boundary: you either respect it, in which case you never cross it, or you don't, in which case you are ethically culpable.

I have previously argued that the fact that we work on the boundary and will frequently be drawn across it means that our registering bodies should design ethical codes that reflect that reality. The unprofessional conduct cannot be defined as crossing a boundary but remaining there (Stokoe, 2020, p. 122). In this final section, I want to consider the extra difficulties that the registering bodies create for any chance to approach an understanding of the truth behind a complaint. This draws upon my experiences both as an advisor or an expert witness in such cases and my experiences in senior management positions in therapeutic organizations charged with the task of managing complaints against my staff or my department. I shall not describe any actual examples for obvious reasons of confidentiality, but I shall draw upon the sorts of cases that would be relevant to the work of the editors of this book. In my experience as manager, I was able to apply two principles. First, turning to the full narrative of a process that has broken down (rather than starting the investigation at the point of breakdown). Second, anticipating that there will be constant activity across the boundaries of the therapeutic engagement, therefore inviting the question, was the clinician actively attempting to maintain his or her professional role or did they allow themselves to move out of a professional role and into something else? Many complaints have merit, but *all* have a meaning. Some are the result of mistakes or even unprofessional conduct by the therapist, some are expressions of the pathology of the patient or else arise from a third party that wants the therapeutic enquiry to be curtailed. In my experience as a manager, it is relatively straightforward to tell the difference and resolve the problem without it ever escalating to an appeal.

It is important to understand that to be the recipient of a complaint is a horribly traumatic experience. First, it is almost always unexpected, so it comes like a sudden assault, shocking and frightening. Secondly, it quickly generates the feeling that the clinician's career might be destroyed. I am aware that a naive assessment of such a reaction would be that, if they are innocent, then they should feel confident about the outcome. This is naive for two reasons that I have already alluded to. Firstly, the shock of the accusation will throw the accused into a paranoid-schizoid state of mind. Massive anxiety always does this, to all of us. It is our default state of mind and I prefer to call it the fundamentalist state because it is a view of the world in which there is a sharp contrast between perfect good and perfect evil, perfect love and perfect hate. Everything is certain and it feels as if there is no need for any kind of thinking (which would be based on a starting point of not knowing). In this state of mind, the accusation that one has done something wrong requires only one of two responses, yes or no. But any good clinician will have accumulated loads of examples of boundary infringements, if they have fully understood this work (that is, being open to unconscious communication), so they will instantly worry that there must be something like that in the background of the complaint. They will imagine that they might be seen as guilty by the black and white judge so powerfully present in this fundamentalist state of mind. It is important to bear in mind that a central feature of trauma, the capacity to symbolize in the emotional and psychological zone of the trauma, is lost. In this way, traumatized soldiers leap for cover when a firework goes off; this is not because the noise is *like* that of the bullets in the traumatic experience, being 'like' something is symbolic. No, it *is* the bullets. Thus, the accused clinician cannot think that past infractions of the boundary are *like* unprofessional conduct, they *are*, or at least will be seen that way by the judge.

The second reason that the view that innocence should protect the accused from such terrors is naive, is that a clinician might feel there is a potential for feeling safe if they felt that their registering body had, a priori, established that the issue of boundary violation is different for psychotherapy work. Sadly, the clinician knows only too well that their registering body has not taken that stand, so, as well as the shock of the unexpected assault, they feel completely alone and exposed.

It is easy to see that, at this point, the traumatized clinician understandably operates from a paranoid-schizoid state of mind. This means that they, like their registering body, will tend towards an absolutist solution to their plight.

If we design the secondary container as a mechanism to provide the best chance to protect treatment of the patient and, if we agree that this will be most likely to be achieved by understanding exactly how the collapse of the therapeutic container occurred, then the first thing to establish is what might be described as the 'personality' of this external container. Lest it sound a bit bizarre to speak about the personality of a system, it is worth saying that writers from the discipline of the psychoanalytically informed approach to organizational consultancy have taken this concept seriously for many years (Jaques, 1951; Stapley, 1996; Armstrong, 2005). Another word for 'personality' might be the 'attitude' of the organization or system. For example, some psychoanalytic training organizations have taken the approach of seeking to avoid accepting those applying for training who they feel are not suitable. The experience for anybody coming to such an institution is very intimidating; they are immediately confronted with an idea that somebody is scrutinizing them to establish whether they are right or not. The alternative is for the institution to welcome interest in their work and application to train; this is expressed in the commitment to receive all who are interested in psychoanalysis and help them to find a place that best fits their skills and interests. The former attitude arises in a paranoid state of mind, the latter from a benign wish to engage and enquire. Thus, the attitude of a secondary container can be defined as a commitment to benign enquiry.

Such an attitude, taken alongside the understanding of boundaries in the psychoanalytic engagement as I described above, is a basis for an effective containment process. The next thing is the understanding that a proper investigation should begin at the start of the therapeutic work, not at the point at which it broke down. The benign enquiry seeks to understand how it came to such a point. Intrinsic to this process will be the understanding that any such enquiry will only come close to the truth if it includes an awareness of unconscious processes, including those taking place within the enquiry itself. In the context of the judicial version of a complaints procedure, one of the most important interventions leads the panel to see how they have been drawn into a dynamic which has been a feature of the therapy. This is central to understanding how it all collapsed.

There are two types of example. In one case the complaint was that the therapist had wrongly charged the patient for sessions which the patient had not attended. The patient's complaint was not only that he had been wrongly charged but that therapy had become impossible because the therapist would not let go of this issue. The therapist's presentation at the panel was high-handed and confrontational. It was clear that the panel were rapidly pushed into an irritated and judgemental attitude towards the therapist. It was only through the process of listening to the patient description of the way that the therapy had proceeded that it became possible to understand what was happening between panel and therapist. The story that emerged was of a therapy in which the therapist seemed to struggle to remember what has been going on and appeared to become more and more rigid in his interpretations. When the panel were freed from their emotional response to the therapist's attitude, they were able to take a more adult and benign approach, understanding that the therapist was suffering from some sort of illness. The panel were able to make a judgement that attended to the disability of the therapist in such a way that the patient also felt understood and was able to consider engaging in a new therapy with a different therapist.

The other example is one in which the complaint, on the surface, sounded very similar; the patient complained that the therapist had changed from being supportive and helpful into being critical and attacking, leaving the patient unable to trust in his therapist or in the process of therapy. The panel seemed very caught up in an idea that they were there to right a wrong. In other words, although they had not noticed it, they had already convicted the therapist. The revelation of the story of the therapy showed a patient with particularly powerful borderline personality characteristics; the beginning of therapy was marked with her continual idealization of the therapist, suddenly brought to an end by a very trivial incident in which the patient felt the therapist had turned into an enemy. The pattern was that these incidents were followed by a return to what might be described as a state of merger with the therapist until there was another incident leading to conflict. The breakdown of the therapy occurred at a point at which the patient had also formed a relationship with a boyfriend. The power of the belief that there really was an attack, a belief that repeated at intervals, suggested that there had been an experience of something abusive early on in the patient's life but that this could only be approached through this form of projection. When the panel were able to see that they were being invited to assume that there *must* have been an abuse, they were able to free themselves sufficiently to make a more dispassionate judgement about what really happened.

The most important point about all of this is that I am convinced that neither of these cases had to go to a panel. If there had been a functioning secondary container at the time of the complaint, I have no doubt that the understanding that I have just described would have been available at the point of the initial enquiry and a containing solution could have been found without putting either party through the agony of this formal, judicial enquiry. These processes are enormously destructive to both patients and therapists and they occur only because the governing bodies of our psychoanalytic institutions will not take a measured, adult and clear stand on behalf of the complex nature of boundaries in the psychoanalytic engagement.

CHAPTER 10

Complaints and incident procedures in the NHS

Romanie Nedergaard-Couchman and Rajnish Attavar

Introduction

Procedures for handling complaints in the NHS are based on a culture of learning from incidents, rather than blaming individuals. The NHS Constitution states 'The NHS commits when mistakes happen to acknowledge them, apologize, explain what went wrong and put things right quickly and effectively.' The NHS aims to have a 'no blame culture' and there is a strong emphasis for individuals and the system to learn from mistakes after they have occurred. Staff members are always encouraged to reflect, engage in supervision and to aim to improve health services. When incidents are being investigated there is a focus on the act (what has happened) rather than the individual (who has done it).

The NHS strives to support a culture of fairness, openness and learning. Staff should feel confident to speak up when things go wrong, rather than fearing blame. In supporting staff to be open about mistakes this allows valuable lessons to be learnt so the same errors can be prevented from being repeated.

Attention is paid to both complaints and compliments. Through the course of a doctor's career, complaints are expected to happen. Clinicians are expected to reflect on complaints or incidents as well as compliments at their yearly appraisal.[1, 2]

The right of the patient to complain is enshrined in the NHS Constitution, hence the processes and policies within the NHS to ensure that any complaints or grievances can be addressed in a timely manner. Various bodies such as the General Medical Council (GMC), the British

Medical Association (BMA), the Medical Defence Union (MDU), the Medical Protection Society (MPS) and local NHS organization support the professional dealing with any complaints.

NHS procedures for complaints and incident investigations

In the NHS various bodies are in place which look at professional registration, maintaining good clinical practice, indemnity and complaints, such as the relevant unions (British Medical Association and UNISON), in addition to bodies which are semi-independent but are crucial in the processing of complaints (such as the Patient Advisory Liaison Service; 'PALS', see below). These various bodies aim to ensure that the complaints are fairly assessed, investigated and fed back to the complainant within 28 days (most cases are dealt with in this timeframe).

There are also procedural structures in place in the NHS if the complainant is not happy with the outcome of the investigation, for example the complaint could be reviewed by a different set of investigators. The outcomes of serious complaints have oversight of senior Trust executives who must agree with the outcomes of the investigation and if necessary remedial steps can be put in place. This allows the Trust and the person named in the complaint to work in a transparent way to apportion blame to one individual or actions.

Most complaints have multifactorial reasons for the complainant being dissatisfied with the service. The Trust investigators (senior clinical staff) use a tool called Root Cause Analysis (RCA), to look at why the complaint occurred and what learning could be gained from the investigation. Elements such as patient factors, environmental factors, professional factors, waiting lists, communication factors and others may be investigated, to form a complete systemic review of the problem. The review also includes an Action Plan, which describes how best to support the service and the individual moving forward.

In rare conditions a complaint may well proceed to disciplinary action during which time the staff who are in the disciplinary process would be able to access support from either their own union or from their personal indemnity provider (Medical Defence Union or Medical Protection Society for medical professionals) to defend themselves against the allegation. The disciplinary process could be either local within the organization or in serious breaches could well be held by the licensing authority such as the General Medical Council for Doctors or the Nursing and Midwifery Council. Both these bodies are independent of the complainant, the complaint and the employing NHS Trust. Hence it is believed that this process would allow a fair hearing and outcomes.

In extremely rare circumstances there may be a judicial review in the outcomes of complaint, or the care given to a patient. A judicial review is usually requested by the Secretary of Health or when all procedures have been exhausted and the complainant could request a judicial review into the process.

Complaints in the NHS follow a path where there are options to address the need or to look at complaints in an unbiased way before it proceeds towards disciplinary or goes in front of the licensing authority. Most complaints within the NHS are resolved in the 28 days. This allows for complaints to be addressed within a fixed time frame and in many instances takes the heat off the complained about as the complainant may feel that their grievances have been heard, and remedies for changes to practice put in place. In serious complaints the outcome of the total investigation is usually discussed and there is an open and honest reflection within teams to acknowledge and change practice where necessary. The change of practices may result in safer services for both the complainant and the complained about in the future.

Each complaint made against the department or an individual must be addressed through personal reflections (during annual appraisals which are necessary for the clinician's revalidation). These reflections usually follow on from any complaint or adverse incidents.

The NHS conducts training sessions for staff development which have elements on how best to respond to difficult and indigenous patients and on how to seek help within the organization. One example is 'unconscious bias training' which addresses unconscious assumptions all staff can make. In most instances large organizations do not blame the patient for the complaint even if those complaints are multiple in number.

For patients who have not had a satisfactory outcome for the complaints and have raised these issues through the local MPs or anonymously, the complaint can be considered by two governing bodies (professional bodies such as the GMC, or regulatory bodies such as the Care Quality Commission). In most instances these bodies ask the local

NHS Trust to relook at the complaint, and report back to them and the complainant.

The NHS complaints process requires a clear separation of complaints from disciplinary action. Where a decision is made to embark upon a disciplinary investigation, action under the complaints procedure on any matter which is the subject of that investigation must stop. Where there are aspects of the complaint not covered by the disciplinary investigation, they may continue to be dealt with under the complaints procedure. A similar approach is adopted in a case referred to the GMC.

If a complainant asks to be informed of the outcome of the disciplinary investigation, they will generally be given the same information as if the matter had been dealt with under the complaints procedure – what happened, why it happened and what action has been taken to prevent it happening again. They can also be told, in general terms, that disciplinary action may be taken because of the complaint.

Patient Advice and Liaison Service

NHS hospitals and Trusts have a service called Patient Advice and Liaison Service, 'PALS', which initially handles complaints or queries from patients. The PALS offers confidential advice, support and information on health-related matters. They provide a point of contact for patients, their families and their carers. The team will liaise with the clinical teams and aims to resolve any issues immediately, if possible. PALS aims to help resolve concerns or problems for patients using the NHS and can give information on how to get independent help if they want to make a complaint. PALS aims to help improve NHS services based on concerns and suggestions from patients. Patients can make complaints to PALS.[3] Alternatively complaints can be made to the commissioner of the hospital: either NHS England or the area clinical commissioning group (CCG).

Root Cause Analysis

The Root Cause Analysis tool kit (RCA) is an investigating and analysis framework used in the NHS to identify contributory, influencing or causal factors that contributed to the incident (Dineen, 2002).

When a complaint is made within the NHS this is usually investigated through a process called Root Cause Analysis, as it is identified that there is not one single cause for an incident to occur, it is likely that there are several factors some of which are contributory or causal factors which may be highly specific to the incident. Alternatively there could be an environmental or working ethos within the system which has led to the incident.

The incident is usually reviewed under the following categories:

- **Patient factors**: Those unique factors in a patient, for example existing comorbidity or mental illness, which may have played a significant factor in the incident.
- **Individual factors**: This could include psychological factors, working relationship factors which may also have played a role in the incident.
- **Task factors**: These are unique support structures which help clinicians deliver a particular task (therapy or clinical procedure).
- **Communication factors**: There could be other factors which could result in miscommunication, either verbal or non-verbal, which may have led to the incident.
- **Team and social factors**: Environmentally there could be team and social factors, for example how well the team works and how the individual relates to the management structures within the team. Supervision or support from a supervisor or manager during the incident could be crucial.
- **Poor working conditions**: This could include noise, building work, overcrowding or poor lighting which in some instances could lead to incidents or complaints.
- **Educational or training factors**: Lack of appropriately trained personnel able to do the task assigned to them could well play a part.

All these systemic, individual and training factors for an incident or a complaint to have occurred will be looked at during the RCA. When these factors are collated at the end of the investigation, they are assigned in a diagrammatic fashion, for example a fishbone diagram, to show how different causative factors may have led to or may be related to the incident.

144 THE PSYCHOTHERAPIST AND THE PROFESSIONAL COMPLAINT

The RCA is helpful in looking at multiple factors which may all have led to an incident occurring, it is looked at in the process of no blame culture within the NHS so that different factors could be improved to prevent similar incidents occurring in the future.

Tips on handling a complaint

The Medical Protection Society notes some advice on how to handle a complaint:

1. Make sure you understand exactly what the complaint is about – don't attempt to offer any explanation until you're sure you know what happened.
2. Maintain an empathetic and professional attitude throughout.
3. Don't be slow to apologize if a deficiency in care has occurred (acknowledgement and apology for shortfalls in care prevent many more claims than stonewalling and prevarication).
4. Be open and straightforward – cagey or evasive answers are a sure way to make complainants suspicious that they are not being told the whole truth.
5. In complaints processes, as in any part of professional practice, patient confidentiality should be maintained, and confidential information not disclosed unless you have the appropriate authority to do so.
6. Tell the complainant how the process works, who the contact person at the trust will be and how long it is likely to be before the trust will be in contact with them. Current regulations state that the complaint must be acknowledged within three working days of receipt, at which time the trust should agree a time frame with the complainant.
7. If, as a result of the complaint, action is taken to avoid the same thing happening to someone else, tell the complainant – it's often one of their prime concerns.[4]

A patient making multiple complaints

Some patients may make several complaints. Within the NHS each complaint is taken on its own merits and is usually investigated in its fullness; regardless of previous complaints each complaint is seen separately.

Even if multiple complaints have been found to be inaccurate, any new complaint would not be prejudiced by previous multiple complaints by the same patient. Sometimes patients would seek therapy or clinical support from a different clinician if there are difficult relationships between the patient and therapist. In these scenarios a large organization (most psychiatry and psychotherapy services have got multiple professionals) can be able to take on the patient who made a complaint against therapist. In some instances, this may be successful in managing expectations and reducing dissatisfaction with the therapist or therapy. In some instances patients are not seen on their own with a single therapist; there may be two therapists (one male and one female) during any clinical work with the patient especially if the patient has a history of insecure or enmeshed attachments which may then lead to complaints against a therapist. (Defensive practice can be the preferred route in some instances.)

Complaint investigations leading to suicides amongst doctors

In 2014 a review was published on doctors who had committed suicide while under GMC fitness to practise investigations. The review identified 114 doctors who had died during the period 2005 to 2013 and had an open and disclosed GMC case at the time of death (Horsfall, 2014). The purpose of the review was to examine the GMC's processes in order to make any possible improvements to reduce the impact of investigations on vulnerable doctors and prevent suicide as a result of these investigations. There had been 28 cases of a doctor committing suicide or suspected suicide while under investigation during this period. Many of the suicides were committed where the doctor suffered from recognized mental disorders, such as depressive illness, bipolar disorder and personality disorder, with a number also suffering from drug or alcohol addiction. Among other factors that may also have affected the suicides were marriage breakdown, financial hardship, the involvement of the police and the impact of the GMC investigation.

The following recommendations were made:

1. Doctors under investigation should feel they are treated as 'innocent until proven guilty'.
2. Reduce the number of health examiners' reports required for health assessments.
3. Appoint a senior medical officer within the GMC to be responsible for overseeing health cases.
4. Introduce case conferencing for all health and performance cases.
5. Set out pre-qualification criteria for referrals from NHS providers and independent employers.
6. Make emotional resilience training an integral part of the medical curriculum.
7. Expose GMC investigation staff to frontline clinical practice.
8. Develop a GMC employee training package to increase staff awareness of mental health issues.

Recommendations for GMC stakeholders:

9. Establish a National Support Service (NSS) for doctors[5]

Clinical case scenario 1

This case scenario is amalgamated from a variety of clinical experiences.

Becky was a 29-year-old lady who had weekly appointments with her psychiatrist, due to longstanding difficulties with low mood, anxiety and traumatic experiences in her childhood. One day, Becky had woken up after a bad night sleep because the neighbours had a party which kept her up all night. Despite feeling tired and with a slight headache she decided to make it to her appointment anyway. Due to an accident the traffic on the way to the hospital was very bad and the weather was terrible. When Becky arrived at the hospital she was later than usual and all the car park spaces were taken. Becky drove around the local neighbourhood to find a space to park, and eventually parked in a residential street. After she had parked she had to walk for ten minutes through the pouring rain. 'Why does a hospital not provide sufficient parking spaces for their patients?' she grumbled.

Becky mentioned her name when she arrived at reception. The receptionist initially responded that they had no record of her appointment. 'You must have got the date wrong.' Becky was getting annoyed and said that she met her therapist every week at the same time. The receptionist replied she must have got it wrong. Eventually she looked again and said 'Ooh, Rebecca! I see it now.' Becky's name on patient records was Rebecca, but she used the name Becky in life.

Becky sat down in the waiting area; it was cold and noisy. Five minutes went by… ten… fifteen… After twenty minutes she asked the receptionist, who said she would check for her. Five minutes later her psychiatrist came in and said, 'I didn't realize you were here, nobody let me know!' The session only lasted for twenty minutes as they started over twenty minutes late. The session was challenging and Becky did not feel like talking, she felt angry. Her psychiatrist looked bored and tired and seemed distracted. Becky was feeling angry and frustrated. It seemed the psychiatrist did not even care what she was saying to him, why was she even there? She had asked for medication many times but he never gave her a prescription! Also he kept telling her she had a personality disorder, which she did not agree with; she felt she suffered from depression.

After Becky left her appointment she had to walk another ten minutes through the pouring rain, then found her car with a ticket on it for being parked in the wrong place. At this point she was feeling furious, had a bad headache and felt this was all very unfair. She was trying her best to get help, why was everybody treating her so badly?!

Becky wrote a letter of complaint to the hospital.

'First of all, my name is Becky as I have explained to this hospital about a hundred times!' She complained about the lack of parking spaces at the hospital, about the receptionist not knowing what she is doing, her psychiatrist being twenty minutes late, and then just receiving a generally rubbish service with a terrible psychiatrist! She wrote that her diagnosis was wrong (she does not have a personality disorder) and all she needed was medication, which they were refusing to give her. She ended by saying, 'My psychiatrist must be the worst psychiatrist in this country, working in the most patient-unfriendly hospital!'

The complaint arrived at PALS, the Patient Advice and Liaison Service, at the hospital. The team contacted the psychiatrist to inform him about the complaint. They discussed the information which was described in the complaint. The PALS team then contacted Becky and offered her an appointment with her psychiatrist to discuss her concerns.

A week later Becky had a meeting with her psychiatrist. This time, fortunately she got to the hospital on time and was able to find a parking space. The regular receptionist, who knew Becky, was back at work and greeted her when she came in. Her psychiatrist was on time for the appointment.

Becky and her psychiatrist discussed Becky's grievances in detail and her psychiatrist apologized to her. He told her he would make sure her patient records clearly state that she is called 'Becky' instead of 'Rebecca'. The receptionist that week was temporary as the regular receptionist was on holiday. The psychiatrist explained they would make sure receptionists receive adequate induction and training. They also talked about her difficulties and how psychological therapy would probably be more beneficial for her in the longer term than medication. Becky left feeling satisfied. The complaint did not need to be raised any further.

Clinical case scenario 2

This case scenario is amalgamated from a variety of clinical experiences.

Mandy was a 33-year-old lady with borderline personality disorder and a long history of self-harming behaviour and several suicide attempts. She had been admitted to psychiatric hospitals several times, which had proven to be unhelpful. While Mandy was on the ward, her self-harming behaviours would escalate, she would not engage with treatment, she had used alcohol and drugs, tried to abscond, she had become aggressive towards staff and started a relationship with another patient in the hospital.

Mandy was living in a flat on her own, with support from a psychiatric nurse from the community team who met with her regularly, as well as reviews with her psychiatrist. She also had sessions with a psychotherapist. The general approach agreed by the multidisciplinary team was that admission to inpatient hospitals were unhelpful for Mandy.

The duty psychiatrist was on call in the accident and emergency department (A&E) of the hospital that night. He had had a very busy few weeks with lots of demands and felt tired and drained. He was finding it especially difficult to deal with patients with personality disorders, as he knew the right treatment would be psychotherapy but there was a long waiting list for patients to start treatment. Several of his patients had been self-harming and he was finding it emotionally difficult to deal with this patient group.

The duty psychiatrist received a call about Mandy at 2 a.m. She had presented to A&E, after she told her psychiatric nurse she had taken an overdose of her medication. Her psychiatric nurse advised her to go to A&E. Mandy was demanding an admission to hospital. After reading her patient notes, the duty psychiatrist was aware of her diagnosis and that the general advice for her was that inpatient admissions were unhelpful.

Mandy met with the duty psychiatrist for an assessment. She was agitated and feeling anxious. She was worried about her ongoing thoughts of suicide and was requesting that she was admitted to hospital to ensure her safety. The duty psychiatrist explained to her that it would be more helpful for her to go home, and receive follow-up from her community mental health team. Mandy was becoming more and more agitated and felt that this psychiatrist was not interested in her and not wanting to help her. She felt he was judging her due to her diagnosis of personality disorder.

After being sent home, a few hours later Mandy presented to A&E again after having taken another overdose of medication and self-harmed by cutting her legs. She was assessed by a different psychiatrist who decided to admit her to hospital for a brief period of time.

Mandy made a complaint about the duty psychiatrist to the hospital. She wrote that she felt he had a prejudice against people with personality disorders. Mandy said that he did not treat her fairly and did not listen to her, because she had a label of personality disorder. Mandy described that he 'could have killed her' as he sent her home that night. She said 'my blood is on his hands' and that he should be 'struck off' from the Medical Register. Mandy stated that the psychiatrist did not treat her well and had no interest in her. She wrote that the psychiatrist had already made his mind up about her, before he walked in to the room.

The complaint went through PALS and an investigation was organized. Senior clinical members of the hospital completed the investigation and concluded that the duty psychiatrist had not made any errors. This decision was based on a reasonable balance of probability: it was deemed that it was more probable than not that the psychiatrist had not made any errors. At the time of the meeting, with the information he had at hand, the psychiatrist was deemed to have made a careful consideration, taking into account different factors. In the situation he was presented with, it was decided he made a reasonable decision at the time.

When the outcome of the complaint investigations came back to

Mandy, she was very unhappy. She wrote to her MP and threatened to write to the newspapers. She felt she had been discriminated against due to her diagnosis of personality disorder. However, the Trust reviewed the complaint investigation and remained of the opinion that there was no evidence of wrongdoing from the psychiatrist.

Conclusion

In the NHS there is a general culture and desire to avoid being punitive when it comes to complaints. Investigations into complaints focus on the system and different factors which may have played a part; rather than blaming an individual, aiming to find any issues within the system and not focusing on one person. The root causes which are investigated are varied and include environmental factors, personal factors, work factors and training. The aim is to be a system of enquiry, trying to find ways of improving services to make them better in the future.

There are various differences between psychiatrists working within the system of the NHS and psychodynamic psychotherapists working independently. Within the NHS, a psychiatrist or psychologist may provide short-term sessions such as six to twelve sessions of cognitive behavioural therapy. The therapist would be working within a multidisciplinary team and there would be the possibility to change therapists if required. This is in contrast to an independent psychodynamic psychotherapist who may work with one client for a long time, doing one to one sessions.

In the NHS different levels exist between the patient, the therapist, the multidisciplinary team, management and overarching organizations. A complaint in the NHS will go through the PALS team, management in the hospital; there would be a root cause analysis by separate, independent managers in the Trust. This is different from the individual relationship a psychodynamic psychotherapist might have with their client.

Within the NHS, if a complaint is made, there would need to be real evidence of wrongdoing from the psychiatrist before anything would be escalated to regulating bodies. The registration body, such as the GMC for doctors, would not be involved unless there was evidence of actual wrongdoing from the doctor. The systems set up in the NHS for monitoring the conduct of doctors and investigating any complaints have various layers and independent organizations to investigate, with a general vision to improve services and look into any causes within the system that could be addressed and improved.

Notes

1. NHS improvement: www.england.nhs.uk/patient-safety/a-just-culture-guide (accessed 3 July 2022).
2. Hertfordshire Partnership University NHS Foundation Trust complaints training.
3. www.nhs.uk/nhs-services/hospitals/what-is-pals-patient-advice-and-liaison-service/ – What is PALS (Patient Advice and Liaison Service)? (accessed 3 July 2022).
4. Medical Protection Society: www.medicalprotection.org/uk/articles/dealing-with-complaints (accessed 3 July 2022).
5. www.gmc-uk.org/-/media/documents/Internal_review_into_suicide_in_FTP_processes.pdf_59088696.pdf (accessed 3 July 2022).

CHAPTER 11

Uses, misuses and abuses of fitness to practise processes

Philip Cox

All psychotherapy accrediting bodies lay claim to protecting the public. However, there is some evidence from the literature and experiential case studies that when misused, Fitness to Practise (FtP) processes can put members of the public, as well as psychotherapists, counsellors and psychologists (hereon therapists), at risk of harm. The topic of the uses, misuses and abuses of FtP processes is rarely discussed by the accrediting bodies, in trainings or openly among therapists. Philosophically, I suggest we are all sometimes the good and the bad therapist (Shohet, 2017). In delivering or receiving psychotherapy, likely every psychotherapist has experienced the often delicate tension between good and less than good therapeutic practice.

This chapter explores three key questions: are our accrediting bodies (who register, accredit and regulate us as professionals) unintentionally supporting misuses of FtP processes; how far are our accrediting bodies facilitating intended abuses of FtP processes; and are our accrediting bodies there to protect their members, and also the public, from the misuses or even abuses of FtP processes.

Theoretical grounding of the uses, misuses and abuses of FtP processes

The theoretical grounding underpinning this exploration of psychotherapists' experiences of FtP processes, is Merton's (1936, 1972) theory of the unanticipated (also known as unintended) consequences of purposive social action. I employ the theory to explore the dilemmas that emerge when the unintended consequences of actions expected to protect the public result in an unintended or unexpected negative outcome. Each of the five cases below highlights and explores a different aspect of unintended harm through the lens of a different use, misuse or abuse of a FtP process. The aim is to consider what we can learn from FtP processes that sometimes fail to meet the intended aim of protecting the public, and to educate all the stakeholders in order to limit unintended harm.

Prevalence

Fonagy (2012) proposes that iatrogenesis (unintended harm engendered by a therapist or a social system) is the most pressing under-researched and under-reported phenomenon in psychotherapy today. Reports of unintended harm in the therapeutic relationship range from 'does not exist' or 'so small it does not merit exploration' (non-significant in House, 2008; 2 per cent in Fleischer and Wissler, 1985), to 5–6 per cent (Clark, 2016), to 27 per cent (Williams, Coyle and Lyons, 1999). Across the literature, the most commonly reported figure of unintended harm hovers around the 10 per cent mark (Barlow, 2010). Therefore, the effect size for psychotherapy outcome in the negative direction is here applied at a conservative benchmark figure of 10 per cent. The phenomenon of unintended harm is reported in the literature irrespective of nationality, therapeutic modality, therapeutic setting or research methodology applied (Cox, 2017a).

For a conceptual consistency across the cases, harm is defined as, 'a negative effect [that] must be relatively lasting, which excludes from consideration transient effects and must be directly attributable to, or a function of, the character or quality of the experience or intervention' (Strupp, Hadley and Gomes-Schwartz, 1977, pp. 91–92). The term accrediting body refers to an organization that accredits and registers a psychotherapist, while the term regulatory refers to the actual FtP process, which may be managed by an independent arm of the accreditation body. Misuse is defined as using something in an unsuitable way or in a way that was not intended (unintended: Cambridge Dictionary, 2021a). Abuse is defined as using something for the wrong purpose in a way that is harmful or ethically wrong (Cambridge Dictionary, 2021b). This includes psychological and emotional abuse, defined as the use of intimidation, coercion, harassment, use of threats, humiliation, bullying and unjust practices (Social Care, 2020).

Complaint numbers

Across the accrediting bodies, the most common causes of complaints are almost invariably: failure to set and maintain professional boundaries with a patient; breach of patient confidentiality; and dissatisfaction with the manner in which the Registrant provided therapy (Cox, 2017b). Each year, the Professional Standards Authority (PSA) audits the statutory and voluntary holders of professional accreditation registers. These audits enable a comparison of the professional bodies' FtP processes.

National Counselling Society (NCS) and National Hypnotherapy Society (NHS)

In 2019–20, the combined NCS and NHS registers had 9000 members, and actioned 12 complaints. Four complaints progressed to full Panel hearings. This means 0.13 per cent of the membership had concerns raised about their FtP (PSA, 2020).

British Association for Counselling and Psychotherapy (BACP)

In 2020, the BACP register had 57,000 members of all grades (BACP, 2021a). BACP received 191 complaints of which 129 became cases. This means 0.34 per cent of the membership had concerns raised about their FtP. Of the 116 Investigation and Assessment Committee (IAC) assessments, 42 complaints were dismissed, 18 complaints were referred to a higher level disciplinary hearing and 24 had no case to answer.

The British Psychoanalytic Council (BPC)

As of October 2020, there were 1690 members on BPC's register (PSA, 2021a). The BPC received six complaints against Registrants, two of which progressed to Practice Reviews and four which were progressed to the more serious full Panel hearings. Therefore, 0.35 per cent of the membership had concerns raised about their FtP.

Health and Care Professions Council (HCPC)

In 2020, the HCPC (2020) register had 24,290 practitioner psychologist members. The HCPC received 175 complaints concerning practitioner psychologists, which means 0.72 per cent had concerns raised about their FtP.

United Kingdom Council of Psychotherapy (UKCP)

In October 2020, the UKCP register had 8455 full clinical members (PSA, 2021b). In 2019–20, UKCP received 86 formal complaints (PSA, 2021b). Forty-eight complaints were investigated under UKCP's formal Complaints and Conduct Process, eight of which were referred to an Adjudication Panel. This means 0.78 per cent of the membership had concerns raised about their FtP.

British Psychological Society (BPS)

The BPS shows the impact of such statistics. It acknowledges that 'whilst the volume of complaints may appear small in number, this year has seen a trend for the potential misuse of the complaints process. The complaints related mainly to personal conduct between Society members rather than FtP. The volume of complaints is a strategic risk for the BPS and was considered at the Risk Committee. It would be valuable for a regular complaints report to help identify trends and themes' (BPS, 2020, pp. 5–6). The BPS's draft Member Conduct Rules has recently been sent to members to 'stress test' the rules against a range of scenarios. The aim is to improve informal resolution and to reduce misuses of the procedure.

The burden of current fitness to practise processes

In 2015, the average cost per case of HCPC (2015) FtP processes at the initial stage was £5439; and at full Panel hearings was £33,403. The overall average cost per case was £9228. The HCPC (2015, Foreword) acknowledges, 'we know that there are significant differences between the accrediting bodies and the FtP research seeks to help identify some of the reasons behind these differences, and suggest ways in which costs may be reduced further in the future'. Across the accrediting bodies, the majority of the fees charged to members are dispensed for concerns about a tiny proportion of members. In 2018, 45 per cent of the total HCPC budget was spent on FtP cases (HCPC, 2018). Given the numbers of Registrants acquitted at full Panel hearings, I suggest that one way to reduce costs significantly is through a threshold test that is fit for purpose vis-à-vis the uses, misuses and abuses of FtP processes.

Subsets within the data of misuse and abuse cases

While the number of Registrants who have had a formal complaint made against them is statistically small, the statistics obscure a subset where FtP processes are unintentionally misused. The misuse can be enacted by the Complainant or the accrediting body. Indeed, the PSA acknowledges the 'number of cases which go through the process resulting in a decision to take no further action is too high, and patients and the public can feel disenfranchised from the process' (PSA, 2016, p. 9). Yet there is a deeper hidden subset; people who experience an intentional abuse of a FtP process by a registered psychotherapist. The PSA recognizes 'the under-prosecution in a number of cases' (PSA, 2016, p. 11). It is these subsets of the misuses and abuses of FtP processes that is the focus of this chapter.

Complaint categories and the threshold test

Whilst the approach to FtP investigations is not identical for all the regulatory arms (here on the regulatory body) of the accrediting bodies, the threshold test also known as the Realistic Prospect Test, is similar. In effect, 'We have a threshold policy to help us to identify those cases that raise a FtP concern and require investigation. It supports our core purpose of maintaining public protection by enabling us to make decisions that are fair, transparent and consistent, while at the same time allowing us to manage our resources effectively' (HCPC, 2019, p. 1).

Complications with the threshold test

Two regulatory bodies, the HCPC and the BACP, have published enough data to assess complications with the threshold test. The HCPC considers its data 'appears to show that the threshold policy is operating as intended as fewer cases are being closed by staff and more cases are being considered by the ICP (Investigating Committee Panel), which is independent of the HCPC' (HCPC, 2020, p. 28). However, the HCPC states the data shows that 31 per cent of the cases considered at its final hearings (across all its Registrants) were not well founded (HCPC, 2019, p. 12). This means that nearly one-third of cases passed the threshold test, and then passed the ICP stage, and then the Registrant appeared before a full disciplinary Panel before being cleared.

The claim that the threshold policy is operating as intended because fewer cases are being closed by staff, and more cases are being considered by the ICP, is deeply flawed. While the HCPC's complaint trend (and across the accrediting bodies) is upwards, the HCPC's trend to close cases early is downwards. Further, that 31 per cent of the Registrants are eventually cleared of any wrongdoing, adds to my concern that an unknown number of Registrants are vulnerable to malicious complaints. My concern is encapsulated by, the 'statistical information available to us shows that a greater proportion of complaints are proceeding through the HCPC's fitness to practise process' (HCPC, 2020, p. 28). It seems a false equivalence to believe that the progression of a greater proportion of complaints means the FtP process is working; I suggest it actually demonstrates that the process is failing to protect the public, the Registrants and the reputation of the accrediting bodies.

We can assess the data published by another accrediting body, the BACP. The BACP's Public Protection Committee's (PPC) strategy includes: effective regulation and commitment to quality assurance; and the effective and efficient delivery to meet public protection needs and make optimum use of available resources. The PPC reports of '116 IACs held in 2020, 42 complaints were dismissed' (BACP, 2021a). This represents 36 per cent of cases, which is similar to the HCPC's 31 per cent. My analysis of the data indicates that of the more serious complaints sent to the IAC, 24 per cent of therapists were dismissed. Behind the data sit the narratives of the people who have been though such personal processes.

Introducing the case narrative experiences

This chapter is committed to the patient's need for recourse if they were mistreated by a person they have trusted to help them. This chapter is also committed to the psychotherapists need for recourse if they were mistreated by an accrediting body that they have trusted to act fairly and proportionately with them. It is important to be clear that I am not denying the existence of misconduct but highlighting the misuses or even abuses of FtP processes. Whether it is 36 per cent, 31 per cent or 24 per cent of psychotherapists who have been through a FtP process that was not well-founded, these numbers represent a mismanaged case.

Research: the impact of unintentional misuses of a FtP process

The following section is part of a long-term research project which explores the impact of complaints from multiple perspectives (Cox, 2017a, 2018, 2019, 2020, 2021). For this purpose, I have interviewed many professionals who have been through an FtP process and asked each of them one question: What was your experience of the FtP process? Interviews were transcribed verbatim, and the therapist was invited to comment on the final work. Permission was given to use the personal experiences for publication and all data is fully anonymized. The following narratives explore the unintended misuses of FtP processes across multiple accrediting bodies. The narratives include a Registrant found liable for poor practice; a Registrant found not liable; a case where two psychotherapists facing exactly the same allegations were treated very differently; a complaint against a Registrant holding duel accreditation membership that was managed differently by two accrediting bodies; and one case where a psychotherapist was both a recipient of a complaint as well as a complainant.

Case 1: A complaint is therapy conducted by other means

Context

This case illustrates a full FtP Panel hearing where the organization unintentionally placed the patient at risk of further harm. During an acrimonious divorce, a mother, Mrs Woods (the custodial parent) sought out and found a psychotherapist for her 14-year-old child. The psychotherapist, Mr Brown, was unaware that the father, Mr Woods, with whom the child stayed at weekends, was unaware of his child's psychotherapy. Over ten sessions passed until the father phoned Mr Brown to 'change' the next session date and so confirmed his child was in therapy. Mr Woods visited Mr Brown's practice and an unpleasant exchange took place as the child patient was being collected by Mrs Woods. During sessions, the child had begun to disclose their feelings about the acrimonious divorce and had disclosed witnessing drug and alcohol misuse. This was mentioned during the post-session parent-therapist interaction. Mr Brown was exploring potential safeguarding issues in supervision when Mr Woods submitted a complaint to Mr Brown's accrediting body, which alleged he had breached the child's confidentiality, and mismanaged the post-session verbal exchange. The complainant was not legally represented nor had a supporter with him. The child was not present and the mother was not party to the complaint. I was involved in working with the defendant's solicitor and supporting Mr Brown through the FtP process.

Mr Brown's experience

I invited Mr Brown to tell his narrative of the FtP process. 'The way that they handled my complaint is they literally took me apart – they dismantled me. They didn't see me, and they didn't hear me, and it was almost like umm some kind of horrible pantomime, you know, they allowed my patient's parent to act out his process – that's not to say that there weren't things that I could have done differently, for sure.'

Mr Brown feels aggrieved at the allegation of breaching the patient's confidentiality then being invited to do so by the Chair of the Panel. The Panel was 'allowing a patient's father to question me for about half-an-hour about how I knew about his drug use ... it was just unbelievable. And I turned to my solicitor to say, 'I really need to find some other way of answering this' because, basically, he was trying to make me say that my ex-patient was a liar, and I wasn't prepared to do that. I actually looked at the person chairing the Panel and I said, 'Do I really have to answer this?' Because I was being asked to disclose confidential information to a father, who I knew from his process [during the post-session incident, the bundle and the style of questioning], was going to act that out on my ex-patient. I mean, this isn't keeping the therapeutic space safe. So it was a very antagonistic triad of power dynamics'.

The Panel instructed Mr Brown to respond to the unintentional multiple double binds. Firstly, this patient was Gillick competent (*Gillick v West Norfolk*, 1984). Therefore, Mr Brown is ethically required to maintain confidentiality regarding what happened in the therapeutic space. To disclose such would breach his patient's confidentiality, while breaching confidentiality could be the foundation of a further FtP issue. Secondly, defendants are expected to be open and transparent in their interactions with other professionals, including an FtP Panel. To refuse to answer a Chair's direct instruction to respond could be used to support a finding of unprofessional conduct; to answer could be used to support a finding of unprofessional conduct. From the most serious double bind emerges the ethical 'choice': to answer would likely place the child patient at risk post-hearing when they return home, while not answering places the psychotherapist at professional and emotional risk when they return home.

The case bundle of documents included a report by Mr Brown's supervisor, who noted the deepening patient-therapist therapeutic relationship. The supervisor had identified what seemed to be envy by both parents towards the therapist. 'I mean, it was so obvious to me and my supervisor that this man was acting out his process on me, his wife and their child, yet they [the Panel] allowed that without any intervention to protect the child – they gave a platform and powerful position for a father to act out a damaged early developmental process (Winnicott, 1947) and a very toxic process on us all – and to say to the child: "Look, you know, you trusted him [Mr Brown as the good object father figure] – you shouldn't have done that – come back to daddy." The complaint had developed into 'therapy conducted by other means' (Totton, 2001).

In what Totton (2001) terms a remarkable act of self-mutilation, psychotherapists and by extension sometimes Panel members and regulatory bodies, have amputated their own understanding of psychological processes. The power struggles of therapy (and FtP processes) are what transference and counter-transference are made of. In Mr Brown's narrative, the power struggle shows the point at which the transference and reality met in the disciplinary chamber, in response to 'real' or perceived mistakes, misunderstandings and insensitivities on the part of the psychotherapist, the Panel and the patient's father. In my experience, complaint processes and Panels rarely consider what is or may be going on below the surface (Jacobs, 2001). Particularly where children are involved, Panel members require special expertise, sensitivity and recognition of the absolute need to protect the child.

Reviewing his experience of the process, Mr Brown mused, 'There's lots of shame that's internalized and otherwise from this process, and we internalize the shame of the whole profession.' Mr Brown wondered, 'Well, I'd really like them to consider what their agenda was, what were they hoping for from the complaint.' He suggested the complainant may have been seeking to get 'a leg up' in a parallel process, the acrimonious divorce, in order to obtain full custody of the child. If such was the case, it was undoubtedly a misuse of a FtP process and should have been prevented.

Case 2: A complainant wounded by the complaints process

Context

Mr Smith (the patient) had recently lost his life partner. From the beginning, Mr Smith placed Ms Khan in double binds, which precipitated Ms Khan abruptly terminating the therapy. Mr Smith complained about the sudden, unexpected ending and poor in-session care. Following a full FtP hearing, the complaint was not upheld. Mr Smith had suffered a bereavement, a loss that he could do nothing about; his therapy was killed off and there was nothing he could do to continue it; he then suffered his complaint being denied, a further loss that he could do nothing about. Ms Khan's narrative explores how the FtP process unintentionally engendered serious hurt by compounding the complainant's losses. I suggest the

Panel omitted forward thinking to assess and formulate possible actions if this process unravelled. I supported Ms Khan's solicitor to show the Panel evidence of a pattern of projective identification (an unconscious projection of split off aspects of the self or an internal object which are attributed to an external object (Klein, 1946)) and how this impacted the therapeutic relationship.

Ms Khan's experience

Ms Khan says, 'In terms of the process, how it was acted out is the opposite of protection and well-being. I mean, just how you first get to know that there's been a complaint … the postman leaves a "sign for note" as its too big for a letterbox, and if you miss it you have to collect it. So, there you are in the post office and you think, "What the hell's this?" and open it, while standing alone in the middle of the street somewhere (anxiously laughs). So you're reeling on the spot, saying "WHAT!" Maybe there should be a kind of little letter saying, "Can we arrange a mutual meeting and you can ask questions", but, you know, it's almost like that baggage is thrown over the wall and they walk away without actually wanting to know how it's landed'. In my complaint support experience, receipt of the complaint typically evokes a sense of threat, making it hard to think clearly and coherently. It becomes easy to react with defensive aggression, fearful avoidance, frozen passivity or collapse, which can play out in the disciplinary hearing room (Van der Kolk, 2014).

'The day that we went to the hearing, the way it was set up was the opposite of connection. You know, it was the opposite of kindness. We had lots of cups of tea and biscuits … it's like a courtroom basically. And you're thinking "What's this got to do with this process that they're trying to model [professionalism] – it's almost the opposite. And yet everybody involved in it presumably has a background in therapy. The language used in the documents they sent me was the language of retribution – it's not a language of healing. You know, it's words like lack of moral care, lack of judgement, lack of wisdom, words like that can only be experienced as accusative. And in the process, you start to doubt yourself, you start to wonder if you're properly equipped for counselling, you start to think, "Well, maybe, maybe I am awful. Maybe I can't do this job"'. As Ms Khan observes, 'Well it doesn't align with the code of ethics, you know, it's the one that was used in the allegation, "with care", actually, it wasn't very careful, and it doesn't seem that wise – maybe it would have been different if the allegations were proven!'

'One of the reasons for the "abrupt" ending was that my patient chose not to disclose details about himself, his past, his personal history. He thought this was irrelevant'. Mr Smith had placed Ms Khan in double binds: from her training background, it would be unethical to proceed without more than a name to appropriately assess and formulate a treatment plan, yet to not proceed risked being accused of unethically ignoring the patient's needs and requests. Also, Mr Smith refused to explore declining to engage, or the choices and transference potentially originating in the patient's personal history. Ms Khan recalled that 'Perhaps you [the writer] or my supervisor considered he was effectively "killing me", making me "incompetent" and "nullified" as a therapist – that was, perhaps, the way he felt about his deceased partner. He needed to see how I would respond to being "killed"?'

When I read the original case bundle, I was surprised that the threshold test decision-maker or an investigating committee at an earlier stage, appeared not to have considered the patient picked a female therapist similar to his deceased partner, perhaps to project the pain and hurt from his loss onto and into the therapist and kill her off; and picked a psychotherapist who identified with the confusion and loss. The explanation of projective identification by Ms Khan's solicitor helped the Panel appreciate that without understanding Mr Smith's history or any context for his loss and grieving, and unwilling to practise this way, Ms Khan was limited in recommending more appropriate therapy or counselling. Ms Khan explained to the Panel, 'His insistence in not talking about his personal history severely restricted my ability to offer better support'. Sadly, I consider the regulator supported Mr Smith to harm himself, and Ms Khan and themself. Ms Khan insightfully recognized 'as the patient didn't turn up to the hearing, and didn't communicate that intention to anyone, this was, in some ways, the most painful aspect of the process. In the end he made everyone incompetent, nullified, unable to perform their proper roles; he silenced our voices and took away any possibility of restoration or reparation'.

'The relationship with the patient hasn't finished just because there's a complaint. You know, they're still a person who's suffering, and you still have a relationship with them, it's … it's an enduring bond, isn't it? And we, no matter what's happened, still have to maintain that connection, and they [the accrediting body] don't make it possible to do that'. While achieving a 'good ending' is considered part of good practice, FtP processes inevitably remove this from the patient-therapist interaction. However, the way this case ended with the complaint not upheld, could be understood to mean the patient who was seeking help and support from the accrediting body has been harmed by the very process set up to protect them. This is the antithesis of psychotherapy (Jones, 2001). While Ms Khan was held to account for her perceived actions (by the patient through the accrediting body), we can ask, who holds the accrediting body accountable for their process and actual actions? If the complaint was upheld, Ms Khan feared her name would have appeared on the commonly called 'name and shame' page that the accrediting bodies use to publicize wrongdoing; or, depending upon your perspective, to show how seriously they take public protection (Cox, 2018). In this case, the accrediting body held itself to a very different level of accountability to the psychotherapist. While the accrediting body examines its own conduct and FtP in relative privacy, it examines the psychotherapist's conduct and FtP in public: this is shaming and undermines the safe practice of psychotherapy.

Case 3: Civil disobedience: Identical allegations, different processes

Context

Two HCPC Registrants who self-reported their arrests at the same Extinction Rebellion (Hallam, 2019) climate change event and faced the same allegations, experienced different FtP processes. The information considered here is mostly, if not all, available in the public domain. The HCPC states that it serves to protect the public and maintain confidence in the professions it regulates, and confidence in itself as a regulator. This is achieved by setting professional 'standards of conduct, performance and ethics' and taking action through its FtP process if someone on its Register falls below its Standards (HCPC, 2021). Registrants must follow the law, and make sure that 'your behaviour does not damage the public's confidence in your profession and self-report if you accept a police caution or have been charged with, or found guilty of, a criminal offence' (HCPC, 2021, pp. 7–9).

Dr Jones' and Mr Dring's experiences

Dr Jones and Mr Dring, who both asked not to be anonymized to show solidarity with other health professionals facing FtP processes, did not dispute the facts of their respective HCPC allegations. However, both did dispute that their non-violent civil disobedience action (refusing to move out of the road) at an XR event, impaired their FtP. In a circular reasoning, the HCPC alleged to both: 'as a registered Psychologist your FtP is impaired by reason of misconduct in that: you received a conditional discharge for failing to comply with a condition imposed by a senior police officer under section 14 of the Public Order Act 1986; this constitutes misconduct; and by reason of your misconduct your FtP is impaired'.

Dr Jones' case was considered on-paper by an Investigating Committee Panel, which found she had no case to answer (Jones, 2020). Mr Dring's case was subsequently considered by a full FtP Panel that he had to attend (virtually), which found the allegation was not well founded. The Panel noted that Dr Jones provided information that 2000 health professionals had signed open letters to warn of the risk of widespread trauma associated with climate breakdown. The letters influenced the Panel, which accepted that 'Dr Jones' actions were not regarded by a large number of professionals as bringing the profession into disrepute.'

I argue that once Dr Jones was found to have 'no case to answer', any following case based on the same allegation and with similar mitigating factors should have been reviewed and probably withdrawn. To support my argument, in Mr Dring's case, the Panel noted that his case was strikingly similar to Dr Jones' case. As the HCPC argues that as a responsible accrediting body it cannot intercede in its regulatory Tribunal process (even if there seems an injustice), perhaps there was the option of opening the full Panel hearing with 'we withdraw' our case. Alternatively, within a court procedure, a prosecution may be discontinued where it is clear that there is no longer a realistic prospect of obtaining a conviction (Health and Safety Executive, 2021). To proceed would be a misuse of the process.

Mr Dring submitted that the HCPC's proceedings against him were inconsistent with the actions of other accrediting bodies when dealing with Registrants who engage in non-violent civil disobedience. BACP (2021b) states that in peaceful protests, being arrested would not necessarily bring the profession into disrepute, or lead to withdrawal of membership. UKCP (2021) confirms that in participating in a peaceful protest and charged with a criminal offence, UKCP would only consider matters that call into question suitability to be on its register. The HCPC's (2021) Standards underpin its highly subjective decisions regarding the character of professionals and their suitability to be on its professional accreditation register. In effect, the HCPC has created double binds of its own making as it continues to prosecute cases where there is no realistic prospect of obtaining a conviction. Indeed, the notion of bringing the profession into disrepute is a 'nebulous and highly politicised concept' (Glyde, 2016). The HCPC, which is a statutory regulator, claims to prioritize all cases by serious risk and only the most serious cases are referred to formal FtP hearings' (PSA, 2021c, p. 2). That position is currently untenable. However, a balanced critique must acknowledge that regulation is a learning process and, looking forward, the HCPC seems to recognize the question of proportionality.

In a parallel to the climate emergency, just as our planet has limited resources that we need to use responsibly, the HCPC acknowledges it must manage its register within the resources available to it. Focusing on unrealistic prosecutions diverts resources and attention away from the serious cases. Further, I suggest the HCPC risks tarnishing its own character by differentially managing similar cases of climate change civil disobedience (Cox, 2021). In a curious recent regulatory turn, the Solicitors Regulation Authority was ordered to pay £27,000 over 'heavy handed' tribunal pursuit where the allegations were brought based on what the tribunal called 'errors and misunderstandings' (Hyde, 2021). The Solicitors Disciplinary Tribunal decided to make the regulator pay the defendant's costs after unnecessarily forcing him into a full hearing.

There is no doubt that two strikingly similar cases were processed differently. The HCPC continued to prosecute the allegation against Mr Dring when it became clear there was no longer a realistic prospect of finding he had a case to answer. This amounts to a misuse of the FtP process.

Case 4: 'Burn the witch' – different regulators dispose of a case in very different ways

Context

Mrs Kimathi held professional accreditation with a statutory accrediting body and a non-statutory accrediting body. From the beginning, each of their regulatory arms managed the same complaint in different ways. One struck off their Registrant; the other issued a serious sanction and their Registrant is practising again.

Mrs Kimathi's experience: The first professional body

'I knew I was in the wrong … I knew it. And I was just like, "I'm in deep. I'm inexperienced – I've made a really serious error here, and I know that". And I remember a supervisor at the time saying, "Ring [your accrediting body] because they're not just there to take your money, they're there to support you". So I did, and I was put on a particular FtP process. I'd "self-referred" and they said in this process, if what I said was true it meant me being struck off, but not if it wasn't true – it was frustrating because "Of course it's true because I told you what I've done!" So it just seemed ludicrous to me.' The accrediting body is considering changing this process, yet to date, it remains.

To have such a split process seems the epitome of a black-and-white approach to regulation because there is no flexibility when judging human actions and relationships. Once certain issues are self-referred, the hands of staff are tied by the two options: strike off or no case to answer. 'I felt it was heavy-handed, and not quite what I anticipated from an organization that's in the helping professions – that's not to take away my responsibility but I felt my serious error was quite a complex area that needed some thought and care. And bearing in mind that I'm youngish, and I was right at the beginning of my career, and I had very little practical experience. I was working in a very tricky environment – it was a little bit like "burn the witch" – I felt very punished, um.' Mrs Kimathi was struck off by this accrediting body's register, which meant the case could then be adjudicated by Mrs Kimathi's second accreditation body.

The second professional body

'So with the second accrediting body, because it's a quasi-judicial process, I couldn't face it and I decided not to go. And I thought that was it, I'm walking away from everything, you know. And, to my surprise, that organization didn't throw me out. They said "You weren't here. This is what we decided without you. Can you please come back in a year's time and complete these things? And then we'll make our decision." And I was *really* grateful. I could (pauses) I feel a bit teary talking about it, um, because it just gave me opportunity – what they were asking for was difficult, but not unreasonable … you know, they threw me some rope really and it just felt empathic. I also had a case worker – actually, that's a key difference – I had a case worker and the name of somebody who was, like sharp, no nonsense, but warm. She sort of said, "Don't give in!" Like, "You've apologized, you know, reflected about your situation – this is boding well" – it also gave me a bit of hope and I was able to carry that forward.

'Although I've read some criticisms about the quasi-judicial process, that actually, for me, it meant that it was formal, and done properly and um, I felt listened to actually which was important. And I felt like I was on her caseload, and that was positive. Whereas I didn't feel like I was on anyone's caseload in the other organization. I felt like I was probably in their in tray (gives a little anxious laugh) – yeah, or their out tray (laughs loudly). The thing I've got in my head is [the first accrediting body's regulating arm] were more aggressive because they don't have any teeth – like they *had* to be that way. Yeah, they [the second accrediting body] were willing to sit with stuff that was far more uncomfortable, which *really* surprised me. Yeah, modelling like, "This is how things could be. This is what a professional looks like". It was like they've got the power and they were respectful of how they used it.

'It was painful, the CEO of my now ex-employer organization treated me with real kindness and again, I'm getting teary talking about it – I always felt that in the background they were saying, "We're sorry that we didn't take care of you better… (pauses and sighs) we should have." My employer? They were never held accountable in any sense'. When I asked Mrs Kimathi, 'If someone asked you for advice about FtP processes, what would you say?' 'I maybe would say be careful about which accreditating organizations you register with (gives a tiny laugh)'.

Case 5: Intentional abuse of a complaint process: complaints made by psychotherapists against psychotherapists

Context

While the cases thus far have explored uses and unintended misuses of FtP processes, there is another category that requires consideration; the intentional abuse of a FtP process. More space is given to this case narrative as it raises so many underexplored, under-reported and complex issues that merit exploration. During my years of working with complaints, I have noticed an increasing trend: the number of unfounded complaints for which no real evidence is presented, made by psychotherapists against other psychotherapists, their colleagues. The difference from misuse is that a patient or member of the general public is less likely than a psychotherapist to have awareness of what constitutes appropriate, or inappropriate, professional standards. Also, the psychotherapist has agreed to practise using a code of conduct and has signed up to abide by a code of ethics. The abuse of process falls almost invariably into two groups: psychotherapists seeking to get 'a leg up' in another related process; and 'tit-for-tat' revenge against someone who has made a complaint against the psychotherapist to intentionally trigger an FtP process. The case below explores both. It also explores how the complainant and Registrant switched roles as their complaints processes progressed through multiple organizations.

For reasons of anonymity, the pronouns they and them are used. I have had sight of the original documents, which support the following narrative.

Both parties belong to different accrediting bodies. The complainant, Dr Evans, is a psychotherapist who employed Dr Hall (pseudonyms), also a psychotherapist, to deliver sessions to a range of patients. Dr Evans declined to pay Dr Hall's full salary, initially arguing that the work was inadequate, and arguing subsequently that Dr Hall's inadequacies had placed patients at risk. However, just before making these claims, Dr Evans had confirmed in writing that Dr Hall's work was of a high standard and invited a contract extension. Dr Hall notified the now ex-employer of possible legal action in the small claims court to recover the unpaid salary. In turn, Dr Evans replied that they would lodge a formal complaint with Dr Hall's accrediting body unless Dr Hall stopped 'making threats'.

Dr Hall's experience: The first accrediting body

I suggest it was Dr Evans who threatened Dr Hall with reporting unfounded serious safeguarding issues, if the outstanding salary claim was not dropped. In my opinion, this functioned to 'get a leg up' in any litigation process. Dr Evans did complain to Dr Hall's accrediting body and wrote they would withdraw the complaint if Dr Hall acknowledged not keeping adequate records, which were claimed to have put patients at risk. Once a complaint is submitted for alleged serious safeguarding issues, the complainant may not have the control to just withdraw it. Dr Hall provided documentation (including the records), to show Dr Evans' claims were unfounded. Dr Hall was concerned that any admission to settle the issues would be used to cause reputational damage. To resolve all the issues through an independent third party, Dr Hall commenced litigation.

'Until I told them [the regulatory body] and they asked, Dr Evans didn't say anything about the court case. I was furious that they'd received the complaint and not told me about it, which I challenged them about and said, "you could have interfered with a court process" – so they stopped until the court process was finished'. The complaint handler responded, "We don't usually notify registrants of complaints unless we decide to progress it" to an FtP level. I suggest that good practice across the accrediting bodies, which most bodies apply, is to inform Registrants when a complaint is made and confirm it is being investigated. Curiously, this accrediting body considers 'the complainant must also have given their consent to disclose the complaint to you', which opens the door to misusing the process. Imagine a situation where a patient or employer has submitted a complaint about their psychotherapist, supervisor or employee, and without declaring such continued to work with them. It seems an injustice that one party would know of the complaint and could continue gathering 'evidence' to support their allegations in a subsequent FtP process, and then submit further supplementary evidence. Also, as a psychotherapist, it is ethically incumbent on the complainant to notify the accrediting body that there is parallel litigation involving the same parties. This could alert the accrediting body to the potential misuse or abuse of a complaint procedure by either party. It could also alert the regulatory arm of a potentially malicious complaint so that the body could ensure due process is followed for the protection of all parties.

Litigation

During the court process, Dr Hall told me, 'I felt intimidated by the ludicrous [counterclaim] amount of compensation demanded, which was then more than doubled with no supporting documentation – they were fantasy figures.' Although the regulatory body seemed to show no concern at the submission of misleading and forged documents, the court took a different view: the counterclaim was quickly struck out. Dr Evans then settled the claim in full before it progressed into an open and relatively transparent process in the county court. With the litigation settled, the regulatory body resumed its investigation of Dr Evans' complaint against Dr Hall. Dr Hall said, 'I lost a lot of faith in my regulatory body when they then allowed Dr Evans to submit a second version of the same complaint with information gained from the legal proceedings. And that's when I did the Subject Access Request and saw how Dr Evans was trying to push the regulatory body in a certain direction, towards a full FtP process. All this time Dr Evans had been engineering something around me, and that's when I started to feel much worse because the regulatory body seemed to be buying into it. I was shocked actually – I made them aware his court case had been struck out: and after a year, the investigation didn't pass the regulatory body's threshold test'.

The second accrediting body

Dr Hall submitted a complaint with comprehensive documentation to Dr Evans' accrediting body, seeking a full FtP process to hold Dr Evans accountable for bullying, threats, deliberately maligning a colleague and deception. Of note is that deception is one of the most serious ethical breaches across all regulatory bodies. The regulatory arm sent the case file to a prominent solicitors firm. It is unknown whether the solicitors considered the complaint from a legal perspective (has the law been broken), an ethical perspective (has the ethical code of conduct been breached) or protecting the public. Dr Evans was found to have no case to answer. Of note is that this leading accrediting body has been publicly critiqued for using legal advice which did not focus on public protection.

Protecting the public

By their own definition, the accrediting bodies were 'set up to protect the public and they both really missed it. The court and judge got it immediately – they didn't accept the dubious documents. I'm left with a prevailing sense of disappointment with both of the regulatory processes, but it gives me a lot of faith in our legal system because they weren't having any of it. For me, the most rewarding thing from this experience, if people can learn from it – it's survivable – I felt suicidal at times. Appealing? I don't want to give it any more energy, any more trauma'.

The threshold test revisited

Each regulatory body has its own threshold test (or realistic prospect test) for complaints. Key factors in assessing whether to progress a complaint, and which track a complaint may take, are issues of deception, a pattern of conduct, admissions of mistakes and the level of insight to show learning. The more of these factors that are present and over a prolonged period of time, the more the public are deemed to be at risk from a psychotherapist. In this case, Dr Evans' conduct evidences a pattern to deceptive behaviour across two years and three formal organizations. In my experience of cases where there is misuse of a complaint process, the threshold test is set too low. Here, in this abuse of a complaint process, it was set too high.

I have worked on multiple cases where complainants have intentionally submitted draft documents and parts of documents as though they were the full and truthful originals. The intention was to mislead and engineer a false narrative to trigger an FtP process, in order to achieve a sanction and reputational damage through misusing the accrediting bodies' public 'naming and shaming' of psychotherapists found at fault (Cox, 2017a). However, I cannot recall working on a case where the complainant has provided to three different organizations a substantial amount of misleading or outright false documentation, and faced no FtP process or sanction for their conduct.

This case highlights some crucial issues when considering uses, misuses or even abuses of complaint processes. Firstly, as far as I am aware, there is no sanction for a complainant who submits a malicious or abusive complaint, for instance presenting a narrative that has no supporting evidence or substantially contradicts previously submitted evidence. I was involved in a recent series of malicious complaints submitted by a psychotherapist, none of which were upheld, where defending just one complaint was estimated at £40,000. The organization considered it was less costly to pay a small settlement rather than pay for legal representation. Indeed, sometimes insurance companies will pay a settlement to end a case rather than contest a malicious claim, or seek to protect the reputation of their insured (Kearns, 2011).

Secondly, I suggest a differentiation between patients who complain about their psychotherapist and may re-enact an unconscious developmental process or trauma in or through the sessions, with psychotherapists who consciously submit unfounded, that is unsupported, complaints against another psychotherapist. Currently, it seems both are treated similarly by the regulating bodies (yet not the court), in that there is no sanction or cost for misusing or maliciously abusing an FtP process. The cost of such expensive processes is paid for through membership fees. I suggest we need to open a dialogue for stakeholders to explore how to address malicious complaints by psychotherapists. I suggest further that in cases such as Dr Evans', the accrediting bodies need to be empowered to investigate the complainant. The reason is that a psychotherapist who engages in such long-term and widespread deception may themself be unfit to practise. The accrediting bodies cannot claim the mantle of protecting the public while failing to take action in such cases. I suggest that if the public heard of the facts in this case, there would be questions regarding who is bringing the profession into disrepute.

The impact upon the psychotherapists

The impact of the process upon Mr Brown was profound: 'I got very close to never practising again. I question would I be free enough to work really authentically and congruently and organically with someone to see their wounds? The accrediting body has really shut me down, made me scared to be real in the therapeutic space.' Ms Khan says, 'How has it impacted me as a person – why has nobody asked me that? There must be different ways to peel a banana, you know, restorative justice, the "People most affected by the crime should be able to participate in its resolution". Mr Dring and Dr Jones expressed relief at no case to answer and anger at their accrediting body for trying to control their non-violent civil disobedience. To the first accrediting body, Mrs Kimathi feels 'betrayed'. To the second, she is 'really grateful, for the process and the professionalism that's enabled me to grow as a professional'. Dr Hall said, 'The complainant was allowed to play on fear and misuse psychological tools and information to create fear and panic, to scare me – looking back on it, it feels really abusive – really tormenting me psychologically.'

Of particular interest when considering the mainstream accrediting bodies' approach to regulatory issues is the Bowlby Centre. Its attachment-based approach emphasizes our need for others and the impact on us in later life when early relationships are insecure, dangerous or abandoning. Its first aim is to protect the public from unprofessional or unethical behaviour by any member or trainee. Its second aim is *to protect members and trainees* by the provision of a clear, independent and impartial procedure for the investigation and resolution of allegations of misconduct (Bowlby Centre, 2021: emphasis added). The point is that among all the accrediting bodies, only the Bowlby Centre openly considers protecting the public *and* protecting psychotherapists from uses, misuses and abuses of FtP processes. Perhaps there is a learning here for us all.

Summary

With one notable exception, whatever the outcome of their case, all of the psychotherapists expressed feeling shame, anger and betrayal towards their accrediting bodies. Personally, I was surprised that two psychotherapists expressed a preference for a judicial process, saying it felt safer and fairer than the accrediting bodies' FtP processes. This merits further exploration. It is clear that there are issues of deep concern regarding the FtP processes of all the accrediting bodies. That up to 36 per cent of Registrants are cleared by investigating Panels of any wrongdoing, evidences the system is failing to protect many members of the public and many psychotherapists. This chapter supports that the threshold test can be set too low or too high. There is little in the literature, or transparency from the accrediting bodies, to help us understand the type and level of training delivered to the threshold test decision-makers. How far the test decision-makers can navigate the complex interaction between the quasi-judicial world and the psychotherapy world, such as mapping transferences in complaint processes (Cox and Shohet, 2017), needs further research. I suggest how the threshold test is assessed and applied is the key pivotal point of intervention, and requires further exploration and transparency in order to improve FtP processes, and truly protect the public and those who serve the public.

CHAPTER 12

The Psychotherapy and Counselling Union: therapists supporting therapists through complaints processes – emergent learning and new possibilities for regulatory change

Philip Cox, Richard Bagnall-Oakeley and Sasha Kaplin

Dedicated to Nick Totton, without whom the union and this
chapter would not have come into existence

Complaints in therapy are an intensely emotional experience, typically involving powerful feelings of shame, guilt, anger and fear and often leaving lasting traumatic impact on all those involved. Moreover, most professionals who have faced a complaint, irrespective of whether they were sanctioned or cleared of any wrongdoing, remain fearful of colleagues or the public knowing about their experience. Until the formation of the PCU, such conversations were typically uttered in hushed tones as though complaint processes only involve those bad therapists who are unfit to practise. This chapter describes the development of the trade union for therapists, the Psychotherapy and Counselling Union (PCU, 2017). It focuses on our interventions in the complaints processes of the accrediting bodies, and in supporting our members. We will describe the unique role played by PCU members as therapists supporting other therapists through this complex and emotionally charged procedure. To the best of our knowledge, many of the issues we raise in this chapter rarely feature in the literature.

As a key thread throughout this chapter, we will argue that current complaint processes are often anti-therapeutic and unethical in their treatment of therapists. Further, we challenge the central claim of the accrediting bodies and their regulatory arms that their complaint procedures protect the public. We will scrutinize the inconsistencies and irregularities in the conduct of the current accrediting bodies, as organizational as well as interpersonal processes. We suggest that not only the process, but the concept of 'making a complaint', is fundamentally unsuited to addressing many if not most of the difficulties that can emerge in the therapeutic relationship. We will then suggest alternative models of conflict resolution which we believe could benefit all parties. Please note: the terms 'therapy' and 'therapists' are used throughout the paper as shorthand for the wide range of psychological practices and practitioners.

A union for therapists: the early stages of PCU

Around 2015, discussions among diverse groups of therapists highlighted increasing discontent with our position and conditions as a group of workers, and therapists came together to act. Core grievances included the widespread exploitation of therapists' unpaid labour as trainees on placement and as volunteers, and the increasing dominance of short-term cognitive-oriented interventions in place of explorative relationship-based approaches. There was also widespread concern and anger that therapists' accrediting bodies were failing to adequately support or represent their fee-paying members.

It was felt that, over time, our accrediting bodies have gradually assumed contradictory roles, where they act as prosecutor, judge and jury, which made them focus on 'protecting the public' *from* therapists. This focus neglects entirely their role in protecting, advocating and supporting their members – the therapists. Many of the union's founding members had actively opposed the attempt (during 2008–11) to bring in statutory regulation of psychotherapy and counselling under the then named Health Professions Council. Statutory regulation was seen as potentially restricting and impinging on the therapist's autonomy, which is viewed as fundamental to the therapeutic relationship in virtually all modalities.

Ambivalence and conflict around rules, policies and regulations have played an important role in the union's development. Furthermore, the tensions around the frameworks governing therapists' conduct and the question of whom, if anyone, should have regulatory powers and how these powers are exercised, were highlighted through an exploration of complaints and disciplinary procedures.

In September 2015, 'We need a union!' changed from an expression of grievance amongst therapists to a statement of intent. At the 'Changing the Game' (Psychotherapists and Counsellors for Social Responsibility, 2015) conference in London it was agreed to form a union, and in February 2016 the PCU held its founding conference, elected a Chair – Nick Totton – and an interim executive committee and began collecting membership subscriptions. At first it was not clear what kind of organization this was: were we a 'professional association' like the British Medical Association? Was it possible to have a trade union where most of the members might be (at least partly) self-employed? But many, perhaps most of our members were in precarious, often low paid or unpaid, work, whether in the public or voluntary sector, in private practice, or a mixture of roles. We wanted to move away from the hierarchies, splits and the modality wars of our field, where psychoanalysts, person-centred counsellors and Cognitive-behavioural Therapy (CBT) practitioners too often seemed to inhabit different worlds and speak different languages – we needed to focus on our common ground to defend the ethical foundations of our work. Hence, support for therapists and trainees of all therapeutic modalities quickly became a central aspect of union work. To reflect these competing tensions, the union developed the logo 'Standing up for therapists and therapy'.

Developing our member support work: professional complaints

Over the next five years of sometimes painful and uneven progress, the PCU gradually evolved from a group of three hundred therapists linked by an email list, a constitution, a steering committee and a website, to a formal listed trade union with insurance to cover the union and its representatives. We also began an association with a legal firm (Truth Legal) for specialist advice. There were many developmental challenges:

therapists' healthy tendencies towards creative individuality and autonomy often lead to anxieties – and many arguments! – around structures and policies. Gradually it became clearer what was needed, what was possible – legally and practically, what policies, rules, and structures we required – and what we had the capacity to do. One of PCU's core aims developed into a particularly active area: supporting members facing complaints and disciplinary procedures. In 2015–16, Professor Andrew Samuels had used his professional standing and influence as a former Chair of UKCP to gain some level of recognition for the nascent union from the British Association of Counsellors and Psychotherapists (BACP), the British Psychoanalytic Council (BPC) and the United Kingdom Council for Psychotherapy (UKCP). The first member support cases followed quickly and Dr Phil Cox soon became our lead representative for complaints issues.

Early dilemmas: who should we help?

As our complaints support work developed, multiple dilemmas quickly emerged. There was a consensus that any therapist already engaged in a complaint process could join PCU and be offered immediate support. This accorded with PCU's philosophy, encapsulated in our motto, 'Standing up for therapists and therapy'. But there were dilemmas, too – for example, whether the union would support therapists involved in gross boundary violations such as fraud, sexual or physically aggressive interactions, or acts of discrimination. Such questions revealed the tensions between those who were shaping the formative internal complaint procedure. With no template for establishing a grassroots complaints support network, we were learning *in vivo* through our collective experiences. We agreed that we would offer representation to all members, even those accused of serious boundary violations, as offering 'support' does not imply condoning ethical breaches, but seeking equitable treatment even for therapists who have admitted misconduct or malpractice. However, after heated debates, we decided that we would not accept or represent members practising conversion therapy, and PCU signed the Memorandum of Understanding (Pink Therapy, 2017).

New proposals for regulation

Proposals for the statutory regulation of counselling and psychotherapy have recently re-emerged. The Counsellors and Psychotherapists (Regulation) and Conversion Therapy Bill 2013–14 (House of Commons, 2019) may merge the Professional Standards Authority (PSA), which regulates the holders of Accredited Voluntary Registers (AVRs), with the now named Health and Care Professions Council (HCPC). Each of the professions the HCPC regulate has one or more 'designated titles' which are protected by law. Although PCU has not taken a formal position regarding professional accreditation and regulation, PCU is concerned at the implications of regulation upon issues of power, creative practice and training. The question regarding whether psychotherapy needs to be regulated has its own literature and is beyond the scope of this chapter (for example, Mowbray, 1995; Postle and House, 2009); however, the landscape of regulation is moving rapidly and is impacting complaint procedures. Whether the regulatory status quo is maintained or the proposed changes are enacted, PCU's experiences of complaint processes across the accrediting bodies, voluntary or statutory, suggests the potential changes would not serve to enhance complaint procedures and would be unlikely to further protect the public. We argue that such changes could harm sections of the public.

PCU member support in practice

Since 2016, PCU has been providing support, advice and representation to its members. Early cases were supported on a relatively 'ad hoc' basis, but we now have about 20 member-support volunteers, and a paid member-support co-ordinator. Over time, we have defined three main areas of PCU's support work: complaints processes, which may involve both therapists facing complaints from clients or a third party, and therapists bringing complaints against other therapists or supervisors; difficulties at work or on placements; and difficulties in training such as trainee experiences of unfair or discriminatory treatment by tutors, which are relatively frequent. Occasionally, teaching staff also seek union support for experiences of bullying, exploitation and discriminatory treatment. Our member-support volunteers may bring their own experiences of other organizations, and a few have been trade union representatives elsewhere. Some support volunteers have their own experiences of going through a complaint hearing or disciplinary process – but none of us started with specialist knowledge: the manual for this work has not been written (yet!).

The first step when a member is seeking support is usually contact with the member-support co-ordinator. This may be the first time that the member has spoken to someone supportive about the issues they are facing and, like an initial interview or assessment in therapy, may involve a flood of information and emotion which the co-ordinator has to contain, process and organize, while working out what is to be done. Some cases may go no further than a brief discussion where the therapist can clarify their options. If it seems that further support is needed or wanted, the co-ordinator then asks for a member volunteer to take the case on, and they are put in contact to provide ongoing support as needed. Member-support work involves a unique and unprecedented role, combining emotional support, advice, advocacy and empathy, indeed the 'solidarity' of a fellow worker in the field. Solidarity in this sense implies an intersubjective recognition of the other and their experience, which is necessary for healthy growth (Stern, 2000). Members' testimonies about the support they have received highlights the central importance of feeling understood as well as supported – that a fellow therapist 'gets' the predicament they are in and the context in which difficulties have arisen (PCU, 2021).

Insurance company representatives and lawyers geared towards an adversarial process cannot provide the empathic reflective relationship needed in a situation which can be psychologically, as well as professionally, damaging. The union representative is able to bring empathic relational qualities otherwise missing from the complaints process. However, as well as the emotional labour, there can often be a significant practical workload in the member support task: reading multiple documents and emails, disentangling often confusing narratives, helping to draft letters and seeking specialist advice on specific points. All these hours of work are done, not in office hours with paid time off (as in the traditional established trade union), but when there's an hour between clients, after dinner or at weekends – the development of a dedicated member-support network is a remarkable achievement.

Supporting members does not mean denial of therapist misconduct, or of the client's right to challenge their therapist – our members may also be clients, and we have supported members in raising complaints or grievances against other therapists and supervisors. Also, dedicated support of the member in difficulty does not require a belief that they are wholly in the right. The human realities of fallibility and fragility, shame, self-justification and denial that shape the accounts we hear, mean that we may not know 'all the facts' – we may have to stay with ambiguity and uncertainty about what exactly has happened, or perceived to have happened, to engender the complaint.

Complaint procedures: the therapists' experience

The formal and sometimes quasi-legal language of the disciplinary policy documents sent to a member readily evokes a sense of threat, making it hard to think clearly and coherently. It becomes easy to react with defensive aggression, fearful avoidance, frozen passivity or collapse (Van der Kolk, 2014). All of our members who have faced the complaint procedure say they felt guilty until proven innocent. Therefore, a core part of the member-support role is emotional regulation through listening, offering understanding and validation to enable the 'accused' member to recover their capacity to self-regulate and reflect (Music, 2011).

We found that therapists subject to a complaint typically experience a complete absence of support or even enquiry as to their welfare from their registering body. Following the notification that they are being investigated, there are long periods where the member (who may be unable to discuss their situation with colleagues) is left completely isolated. Members have described waiting many months for Hearing dates which were then rescheduled at short notice, and processes frequently extending for over a year, during which they are likely to be struggling with intense anxiety and shame at being under investigation. Furthermore, in some cases they were prevented from seeing any other clients during this period, which harmed all their other clients as well as their own livelihood – all this regardless of their being guilty or innocent.

When the Hearing does take place, the high standards of ethical, reflective and professional conduct expected of therapists is often lacking from the process, which was commonly conducted like a trial but without the clarity and accountability afforded by a legal framework. We have heard accounts of complaint Hearings taking place in public venues (where it was evident to venue staff who the 'accused' person was), of being left alone in a bare room while the panel members adjourned for lunch, of being sat alone at a table in front of a panel without even a glass of water or a box of tissues. It seemed at times that the ethical standards of compassionate care and attention rightly applied to complainants are sometimes withdrawn from the person facing the complaint. Likewise, although therapists may be asked to write reflective pieces acknowledging their mistakes, unreflective modes of thinking are often applied to inherently ambiguous, complex interactions in a therapy relationship.

A significant number of cases appeared to focus on 'punishing the bad therapist' rather than seeking to understand what had gone wrong in the therapist-client relationship (see Chapter 11). In such cases, the interpersonal dynamics which may have engendered the complaint seemed to be repeated or re-enacted rather than explored or understood. Our support volunteers have witnessed clients' complaints being taken at face value, treated as facts without considering that they may not actually be facts, and may be motivated by the emotional needs of the client rather than by any wrongdoing by the therapist. Testimonies from clinical supervisors, who share responsibility for the therapist's work, were often disregarded. In some cases, panel members seemed to have little relevant specialist knowledge, and a striking insensitivity around issues of sexuality, race, culture, gender-variance and disability, or health issues and working with children have been recorded.

The impact of past trauma and abuse on the client, which may well be a factor in the complaint being made, are often ignored, leading to a process which may become traumatizing in turn for the therapist. We have heard of panels whose members seem unwilling or unable to consider the possible influence of relational dynamics, transference–counter-transference processes or client mental health issues on the rupture in the relationship that has led to a complaint being made. At times the drama triangle was in evidence: the client as victim asks the complaints panel to rescue them from the persecuting therapist, who in turn becomes a victim of the persecutory authorities (Karpman, 2014). Protocols are developed on an assumption that all involved are purely rational beings, so that if we wrote sufficiently comprehensive contracts and followed detailed guidelines and procedures, there could be no grounds for complaints. This illusion leads to focusing on 'which "rule" the therapist has broken', rather than on understanding what had gone wrong in the relationship.

As therapists, we are all aware of the psychological damage done to clients by experiences of shame and humiliation, yet these lessons do not seem to be held in mind by the Hearings process. Members have described feeling 'stripped' and 'abused' by the personal accusations and the hostile tone of the questions they faced in Hearings. We have spoken to a number of members who felt so distressed and disillusioned by disciplinary processes that they were unable to continue working as therapists. We suggest the level of fear and mistrust which many therapists hold towards their registering bodies should be a cause of concern – we hear of therapists avoiding reporting concerns or seeking advice about complex situations in their work, because of fear of the potential consequences for them if an investigation is triggered. We must ask whether this is really protective of the public, or does this adversarial, punitive response to difficulties become a performative denial of the 'shadow' aspects of therapy, therapists and their organizations?

The adversarial nature of complaint procedures

We suggest that current complaint procedures of all the mainstream therapy accrediting bodies, by design or default, engender openly adversarial relationships, which are inappropriate for addressing conflict in the therapeutic space. Based on our collective support-network experiences and the literature (Cox, 2017), we argue that the current complaint procedures inadvertently fan the flames of conflict rather than aim to resolve it (Totton, 2001). Indeed, 'the confrontational nature of proceedings and the stress that hearings engender can affect the health and wellbeing of all concerned ... [and] runs counter to our growing understanding of the situations where things go wrong' (PSA, 2016, p. 1). Rather than an omnipotent fantasy that poor practice, which exists in all professions, can be eradicated, PCU holds a position that we all are 'the good therapist' *and* 'the bad therapist' (Shohet, 2017). We suggest a more appropriate approach is to explore how processes can congruently and consistently support and protect clients, therapists and the public when things go wrong.

The problem of regulation for resolving relational difficulties

Therapy is a relationship and therefore inherently risky. If we feel too unsafe as therapists, we are more likely to practise defensively and be unavailable to our clients. In the wider social frame, there is often an expectation that therapists can deliver fixed, quantitative outcomes and that the therapist can be discarded or complained against if such expectations are not met. Increasing reliance on standardized, manualized approaches which are touted as 'evidence based' may make results more predictable, but it also ignores a wide range of deeper, perhaps more significantly beneficial therapeutic approaches (for example, Wampold and Imel, 2015) while heightening unrealistic expectations in the public.

In addition to standardizing competencies, multiple accrediting bodies have introduced new codes of ethics (for example, BACP, 2018; UKCP, 2019). Proponents argue these changes are essential to protect the public and to keep clients safe from poorly trained or rogue therapists who are considered to present a danger to the public. Superficially, such moves towards competencies and public protection ought not to be a contentious issue for therapists. However, relatively little research has looked at the effects of the ethical dilemmas that can occur when codes of ethics clash with ethical actions (see Chapter 11) and may engender complaints (Cox, 2021).

Where complaints are upheld they almost invariably result in a process of publicly 'naming and shaming' the therapist (Cox, 2018). We argue that if the accrediting bodies' regulatory function fails to meet the standards to which they hold others, such incongruence would underline the need for therapists to have the support of a trade union. Also, we argue that there is incongruence between the public naming and shaming on open websites of therapists found to have made errors, while there is no equivalent open process for the accrediting bodies who have similarly been found to have made an error. The information regarding the conduct of the accrediting bodies in this chapter (and volume), required research time and skills to locate the data and lived narrative accounts, skills that are unavailable to the general public.

The conduct of the key accrediting bodies

The Professional Standards Authority (PSA): the regulators regulator

The PSA is the regulatory body for the UK's ten health and care accrediting bodies (statutory and voluntary accrediting bodies), and is tasked primarily to protect the public. To be accredited, organizations holding such registers must prove that they meet the PSA's demanding Standards for Accredited Registers (the Standards). Health and care accrediting bodies are required to submit fitness to practise (FtP) decisions to the PSA. The PSA has the power to review FtP decisions made by any of the accrediting bodies. The PSA also audits annually a random sample of FtP cases closed by case examiners at the initial stages of the FtP procedure. This is intended to ensure the accrediting bodies are compliant with their own published procedures and that outcomes are consistent. In cases where the PSA has taken a view that a decision is deemed unduly lenient or does not protect the public, the PSA has the power to refer a case to a court of law for a judicial review. In effect, this is an appeal of an FtP decision, and a court has the power to overturn an accrediting body's decision and substitute it with an alternative finding.

The British Psychoanalytic Council (BPC)

In 2015, following the issuing of legal action in the High Court by solicitors acting on behalf of an analyst who claimed the BPC's complaint procedure rules were outmoded, unfair and not fit for purpose (BPC, 2011), the BPC initiated a consultation regarding its procedures. However, while the subsequent changes in procedures resolved some dilemmas, new dilemmas were created. Under the past rules, analysts facing even the most serious of allegations were denied legal representation and the right to cross-question their accuser (Norris, 2015). The PSA's (2021a) most recently published annual review of accreditation of the BPC, directed the BPC to ensure that its website homepage provides more information about its regulatory and complaints handling role. Also, it stated that complainants should not have to present their own case in Practice Review Proceedings (PRP), given their vulnerability. Additionally, the review highlighted a risk that serious matters could be sent to the BPC's PRP, which is a more lenient and more confidential process than other options. Further, the BPC confirmed that what it would publish regarding process outcomes would depend on the specific context of the case. For instance, the BPC will publish sanctions following a full panel Hearing but does not publish interim measures, nor outcomes from the PRP procedure.

The BPC's rationale for this is that such publications might distress the Registrant's other patients, and that it is in those patients' best interests to know as little as possible about their therapist, who is the Registrant. The PSA (2021a) did not accept this rationale, which initially seems at odds with the BPC's key claim to protect the public. However, as the BPC accredits psychoanalytic and psychodynamic psychotherapists rather than counsellors or psychologists, this key difference represents a tension between the model and practice of a psychotherapy accrediting body, with a quasi-legal approach to therapy regulation. PCU has so far not dealt with formal BPC complaints, perhaps due to the relatively small number lodged annually.

United Kingdom Council for Psychotherapy (UKCP)

In 2015, for the first time the PSA suspended a register's accreditation (Jones, 2016). UKCP was deemed not to have met two of the then ten key Standards for accredited register holders: demonstration of its focus on public protection and demonstration that through leadership UKCP shows that its reputation within and outside therapy operates effectively and openly for all stakeholders. In the PSA's (2021b) most recent annual review of UKCP accreditation, UKCP confirmed it is planning to implement a system of 'Consensual Disposal' allowing cases to be closed based on the acceptance of allegations by a Registrant. PCU considers this would greatly help streamline UKCP's complaint process. It came as no surprise to PCU's complaint-support workers that the PSA (2021b) noted a perceived high level of legal intervention to complaints managed by UKCP. Across all of the accrediting bodies, members must carry insurance, and insurers require early notification of a complaint. Therapists are thereby positioned by external forces at the beginning of the complaint process into a quasi-legal defence of their career and reputation. As UKCP noted, legal costs are a drain on resources, which is reflected across all the accrediting bodies. In the previous PSA (2019b) review, UKCP confirmed that it had created detailed guidance on the 'realistic prospect test' (the threshold test) of an allegation being upheld, and had provided training on this to its complaints team and its Professional Conduct Committee – yet the problems persist. Although UKCP is a relatively large accrediting body, relatively few of its complaints progress to a full panel Hearing, which suggests there are multiple ways to avoid full disciplinary hearings and to resolve complaints.

British Association of Counselling and Psychotherapy (BACP)

After a therapist was cleared by UKCP's Adjudication Panel, the client made virtually the same complaint to BACP, with whom the therapist was also accredited. The therapist sought a judicial review, where the judge ruled that to pursue an identical complaint already disposed of by another accrediting body would be unfair, abusive and unlawful (Jones and Norris, 2016). The court determined also that although UKCP and BACP have differently worded ethical standards, they cover the same ground, even if the language used to express them is somewhat different. This confirms that although accrediting bodies may have different ethical codes, how they are applied needs to be consistent across the regulatory arms of these organizations. In 2021, the PSA published its most recent annual review of the BACP (PSA, 2021c). BACP's communications were found to use legalistic language when explaining decisions, and the PSA recommended BACP review its communications with all parties involved in complaints processes, to assure they are appropriate and sensitive to the matters under consideration. The PSA noted concerns about delays in progressing cases where serious allegations had been made, and that there are complaint cases outstanding for 1–2 years. The PSA noted also that there is 'a risk that significant delays may lead to harm and reduce the ability to inspire confidence that the register was being managed effectively' (PSA, 2021c, p. 15). In PCU's experience, these issues are common across the accrediting bodies.

While we acknowledge some of BACP's changes from the PSA's previous (2020a) review support a fairer process such as advisory letters for relatively minor practice issues and agreed Consensual Disposal of cases (which can be questionable), we suggest that while some procedural and justice difficulties were resolved, new difficulties were created. One potential difficulty is the ability of a case manager and Independent Assessment Committee (IAC) to progress complaints without drafting allegations and notifying them to the Registrant. However, the process enables the case manager and the IAC to request written representations from a Registrant. The IAC even has the power to request an interview with the complainant or the Registrant at any procedural stage. This positions therapists who have received a complaint in multiple double binds. For instance, when asked to comment on the complaint and/or be interviewed before any allegations are formally provided, this can provide the case manager with information that ends the investigation. Yet it can also provide information used subsequently to support the complainant when the formal allegations are provided. Where cases drift into the courts, this double bind can become critical as a reparative apology is often presented as an admission of guilt, even though the Care Quality Commission (2021) says the apology required to fulfil the duty of candour does not mean accepting liability. When considering BACP's complaint procedures, it must be noted that BACP holds the largest member register and so unsurprisingly receives the largest number of therapy complaints.

Health and Care Professions Council (HCPC)

The most recent PSA (2021d) performance review of the HCPC found that it is currently only meeting one of the five Standards of Good Regulation regarding its own practice. The PSA continues to report significant performance concerns regarding timeliness, decision making, risk assessments and ensuring parties are supported to participate in the process. The PSA issued the HCPC with learning points that reflect our member's experiences of the HCPC's complaint process, and across the accrediting bodies: poor or unclear written reasoning's for decisions; poor assessment or consideration of misconduct and impairment; and overly complex legal advice and legal advice which did not focus on public protection. The learning points regarding disproportional favouring of the Registrant rather than the HCPC's overarching objective to protect the public, diverges significantly from PCU's experience. This learning point seems inconsistent with the data that the HCPC has a relatively high number (31 per cent) of Registrants cleared of wrongdoing at a full panel Hearing (HCPC, 2019, p. 12). However, it does seem consistent with the PSA's report (PSA, 2021d) that the HCPC did not meet the Standard regarding risk assessments intended to prioritize serious cases and/or progress cases as quickly as possible, which suggests some Registrants involved in more serious cases are disproportionally favoured by the procedural flaws.

The previous PSA report (PSA, 2020b, p. 4) concluded the HCPC's impaired FtP, 'had the potential to undermine public protection and public confidence in the HCPC'. The concerns regarding the HCPC's own FtP parallel many of the concerns the HCPC raises about its Registrants. Further, the lack of consistent disciplinary outcomes across the main accrediting bodies seems reflected in the PSA's 2015 suspension of the UKCP's accreditation for not meeting multiple Standards, yet not with allowing the HCPC to continue investigating complaints despite significant failings for six years consecutively (Jones, 2016). The finding also reflects the PSA's (2021a) criticism of the BPC's questionable public protection decision to not publish some complaint process outcomes as they might distress a Registrant's other patients. From the union's perspective, we note the HCPC has removed the term to become 'the regulator of choice' for all accrediting bodies (PSA, 2021d). However, this seems unlikely to have changed the HCPC's long-term socio-political aim to regulate all therapy accrediting bodies. We are concerned that an accrediting body that fails to consistently meet its own regulatory and FtP standards could be considered an appropriate regulator for all counsellors, psychotherapists and psychologists. We argue that any accrediting body that lays claim to protecting the public yet seems to put at least some of the public at risk, and certainly some therapists by failing to meet its own aims, lacks credibility as an accrediting body or as a regulator of others.

The Professional Standards Authority (PSA): the regulators regulator revisited

The PSA (2020c) has launched a consultation into the future shape of its Accredited Registers programme. This programme provides oversight of a number of registers for health and social care professionals that are not regulated by law. In 2020, the PSA appealed unsuccessfully an HCPC decision (involving a paramedic) regarding its approach to the question of impairment, arguing the HCPC complaint panel had failed to meet the need to maintain public confidence in the profession, and that its determination was insufficient to protect the public interest (Hewitt, 2020a). For balance, the PSA's judicial reviews are generally successful. The judgment helpfully highlights important principles applicable to FtP cases, namely: isolated incidents could show a momentary lapse and may not be reflective of a deep-seated attitude such as discrimination; and a finding of misconduct does not necessarily mean that FtP is impaired (Hewitt, 2020b). The union's support group welcomes the clarification as we have supported and presented cases arguing that a member's momentary lapse of reasonable conduct could be dealt with by a conditions of practice order rather than being suspended or 'struck off' their professional register.

Across the accrediting bodies

The unequivocal *raison d'être* of the organizations accrediting counselling, psychotherapy and psychology is to protect the public. The concerns raised by the regulators' regulator (the PSA) show each of the accrediting organizations is experiencing similar difficulties in managing its register of members, which the PSA evidences is impacting public safety. Across the accrediting bodies, in their quasi-judicial complaint processes, the lack of sufficient procedural safeguards to ensure a fair process is a theme that emerges from the PSA audits of each regulator. This is evident for both the statutory and voluntary holders of accreditation powers. Another theme is the lack of consistency in the outcomes of complaint procedures, where what is considered is a violation of a code of ethics or ethical framework. Within and between each accrediting organization there can be considerable variation regarding what sanction, if any, is applied (see Chapter 11). One particularly concerning inconsistency regards people of colour, who are at risk of facing investigations for lesser perceived practice infractions than their white colleagues, and endure harsher penalties (Cox, 2019); and codes of ethics that largely ignore perceived transgressive sexualities (Cox and Aella, 2020). PCU is collecting data on these important issues, which will be addressed in their own right elsewhere.

A key criterion employed across complaint procedures to assess a complaint, is whether the therapist's action, if known to the public, would be considered as bringing the profession of counselling and psychotherapy into disrepute. We suggest that if the public knew of the issues explored above, to varying degrees the accrediting bodies themselves would be open to public concern of potentially bringing the profession into disrepute. Looking forward, we are also concerned that the HCPC and the PSA seem to be jockeying for position regarding which organization the government may choose, if statutory regulation is enacted, to accredit and regulate the entire field of therapy. Both bodies seem to be looking ahead towards the terms 'counsellor' and 'psychotherapist' becoming licensed or legally protected titles, perhaps as a way to further increase their influence over therapy. As a union, we submit that ostensibly protecting the public is sometimes at the expense of protecting therapists. Philosophically, we propose that to look after the public, we need an organization that looks after therapists: if we fail to look after those who care, how can we look after those who seek care.

The concept of the 'complaint' as the obstacle to change

Totton (2000) argues the biggest obstacle to resolving client-therapist conflicts is the idea of the 'complaint' itself, a construct which is deeply embedded in the psyche of the accrediting bodies. Therapists often work with people who have been failed by key figures at different points in their life. We argue that at times, therapy is bound to involve the re-enactment of such failures. In our collective casework experiences, where the complainant is successful in their complaint, the re-enactment process is reinforced rather than worked with – where the complainant is unsuccessful in their complaint, the re-enactment process is further embedded and expanded in their life rather than worked through. For this key reason, at PCU we suggest that in such circumstances, the accrediting bodies' policing of therapy risks unintentionally harming rather than protecting some clients. Further, therapy and life necessarily involve disappointment, and the regulatory emphasis on grievances can give clients the false impression that disappointment and imperfection are avoidable, and that a complaint procedure can be a solution for their pain and distress (Totton, 2000).

There is rarely room for mediation in a complaint procedure. In our experience, 'once a complaint has been formalized, it has typically become fixed and the parties concerned have become too involved in their feelings and their anger to find a more suitable process' (Palmer Barnes, 1998, p. 94). From our collective experiences of supporting people who bring a complaint, receive a complaint, supervise or train, we need a less polarized process with less rigid positions, to 'help us embrace an understanding, inquiry and process model rather than a right/wrong content model. This may help us work towards all parties being able to voice the feelings, unmet needs, values and expectations which might lie behind a complaint' (Shohet, 2017, p. 71). In PCU's support network, we suggest that complaint procedures mask the accrediting bodies' underlying fears and anxieties, and so the process risks engendering an ever harsher complaints procedure. In the space between the top-down interventions of the accrediting bodies and PCU's grassroots experiences, sits the possibility of Alternative Dispute Resolution.

Alternative Dispute Resolution (ADR)

PCU suggests a therapeutically oriented complaints process could go the route of reflection rather than pursuing an adversarial 'acquitted or sanctioned' or 'right/wrong' process (Shohet, 2017). ADR offers the possibility of a dispute resolution process that can act as a means for disagreeing parties to settle disputes, with the help of a third-party. As an example, UKCP's (2012) ADR process engendered a non-adversarial and reflective process, which any party could leave, with the complaint process resuming from the point reached previously. UKCP trained 40 people to facilitate its ADR process, but the attempt was unsuccessful. UKCP reported that 'nobody wanted it, partly because complainants wanted to bury their therapist and not for them to do it but for others to do it for them' (Pollecoff, private communication, January 2021). This underlines PCU's concern that therapy is bound to involve the re-enactment of a client's past experiences, and that rather than protect the complainant, the complaint process provides a context for the re-enactment process to play out. This resonates with Totton's (2000) view that the biggest obstacle to resolving complaints is the idea of the 'complaint' itself. It also resonates with Palmer Barnes' (1998) comment that once a complaint has been formalized, it typically engenders entrenched positions, and feelings such as anger become too involved.

Promoting a learning culture

The Nursing and Midwifery Council (NMC) has recently produced what may become a 'gold standard' in managing complaints, dispute resolutions and protecting the public. We agree with Philip Graf, Chair of the NMC (2021, p. 2), that 'we are at a turning point for FtP and need to take a new direction to signal a commitment to move away from a blame culture towards a just culture in health and social care'. The NMC and PCU both challenge the assumption that the only or best way to manage complaints is by restricting the practice of therapists deemed to have made errors. In essence, the NMC and PCU propose alternative ways to protect the public, both based on a *learning culture*. In PCU's experience, publicly 'naming and shaming' therapists can be counter-productive. Invariably, those of our members who have experienced a complaint procedure say that whatever the outcome, they practise less creatively, more defensively and tend to no longer work with high-risk clients. Therefore, processes intended to restrict practices rather than enhance learning can have unintended and profound negative implications for all involved.

The NMC's (2021) innovative new approach takes into account the context in which the Registrant was practising when deciding how to manage a complaint. Where the Registrant has been open about what went wrong and can demonstrate what they have learned from it, even where there has been serious harm to a patient, action may not need to be taken. The aim is to encourage Registrants to learn from mistakes and to promote a learning culture, where Registrants feel safe to acknowledge mistakes and learn from them, thereby improving the long-term safety of all stakeholders. Fundamental change is needed to shift from a blaming and fault complaint process to an examining and learning, remediation and resolution process. The NMC (2021) notes that cases so serious that regulatory action needs to be taken are rare. This fits with PCU's experiences and views, and there are criminal proceedings for such transgressions. However, interpersonal processes may be more observable in the more public nursing and midwifery world than in the relatively private world of the therapy consultation room. This means that while the public seems to some extent to be protected from the small minority of such extreme cases, PCU receives complaints, in particular regarding sexual transgressions for which there is little or no direct evidence, yet which leave us concerned about the limits of regulatory action and so public safety. We consider the seriousness of this is often not sufficiently dealt with. We wonder if this sort of case is where the PSA could exercise its power to refer a case to the courts so that a therapist is not only struck from the register, but a legal directive that the therapist does not practise under any name or title can be made.

Funding the resolution processes

The General Medical Council funds a free Doctor Support Service. The support service is independently run by the British Medical Association (BMA) and provides confidential advice and emotional support for doctors going through FtP procedures (BMA, 2021). A key benefit of the service is that 'doctors find it beneficial to have someone to talk to who understands the profession and is not part of the process' (Rowland, 2017). We see the PCU as the body which could play the equivalent role for the therapy professions. Crucially, the BMA funds the support service, which remains independent of its funder. The current complaint system for counsellors, psychotherapists and psychologists is funded through the subscriptions members pay to their accrediting body, that is, their regulator. As the role of the accrediting bodies is focused on supporting the public rather than therapists, the regulatory arms appear to be the wrong institutions for supporting a therapist going through a complaint.

As the number of complaints rises and their complexity increases, along with the use of expensive external legal services, the cost of the proceedings also rises (UNISON, 2021). As proceeding costs rise, so too the cost of membership fees rise. Therefore, we suggest a fundamental change of direction heading towards a less costly and healthier remediation and resolution process. The finances paid to investigate and prosecute complaints could be used to fund a new more therapeutically oriented resolution process. The independent free Doctor Support Service funded by the doctors' regulator provides one model (BMA, 2021). Another model is an Ombudsperson service, whereby the member accrediting bodies forward all complaints to an independent service funded by each accrediting body, who would contribute to a central fund. This could be run by therapists who understand the profession and who are not part of the internal structure of the membership bodies, or the external moves towards regulation.

Conclusion

As we have shown, accrediting bodies and their regulatory arms offer at best limited support for therapeutic learning and reflexivity. They also risk fostering rigidity, defensive practices and unhealthy relationships between therapists, membership accreditation bodies and regulators. We argue that the PCU's emergent model of support work for therapists facing complaints, based on promoting a learning culture regarding mistakes, needs to be incorporated into future regulatory systems. There is an opportunity for the profession to mature and develop beyond adversarial, binary 'good/bad' narratives towards a model of ethical practice which allows for learning from the errors, ruptures and re-enactments that are inevitable in relationship-based work. A relational, learning-based model of regulation would be more congruent with the aims and values of psychotherapy and counselling, and ultimately, we argue, more effective in protecting the public. Through this new, and still evolving development of a trade union for therapists, new possibilities are emergent for reconfiguring therapists' positions in relation to accrediting bodies, regulatory frameworks, and to our clients.

Abbreviations

ADR – Alternative Dispute Resolution
AVR – Accredited Voluntary Registers
BACP – British Association of Counselling and Psychotherapy
BPC – British Psychoanalytic Council
BMA – British Medical Association
HCPC – Health & Care Professions Council
NCS – National Counselling Society
PCSR – Psychotherapists and Counsellors for Social Responsibility
PCU – The Psychotherapy and Counselling Union
PSA – Professional Standards Authority
UKCP – United Kingdom Council for Psychotherapy

CHAPTER 13

Reform

Julie Norris and Andrew Campbell-Tiech

R egulation is a branch of law. Laws that are effective in both theory and practice share certain characteristics. These include accessibility, clarity of purpose, clarity of expression, ease of application and finality. Further, laws should be objectively fair and understood to be so, not only by those directly affected by them but also by the public at large.

As will be seen, the current state of the regulation of therapists[1] reflects none of the above, save perhaps finality.[2] How has this happened?

It usually comes as something of a surprise to those unfamiliar with the world of professional standards that anyone can set themselves up in business as a therapist, analyst or counsellor. There is no legal requirement to belong to one of the professional bodies. There are no educational standards to attain, nor is previous experience required. In short, there is no statutory regulation. In March 2020, Lord Bethel, junior minister at the Department of Health and Social Care, announced on behalf of the government that, despite a number of Private Members' bills seeking to remedy this, there are no plans to introduce a statutory scheme. It is unthinkable that any government would take a similarly relaxed view of the regulation of doctors, nurses, pharmacists or paramedics. If you practise as a doctor but without troubling to obtain the requisite qualifications and authorizations, Pentonville, not Harley Street, awaits you.

The rationale for such laxity is because a large number of therapists subscribe[3] to a voluntary system, the most recent incarnation of which dates from 2012. Through the Professional Standards Authority (PSA), accreditation may then be provided to a professional body, which in turn ensures that its members abide by certain minimum standards.

However, the fissiparous structure of the profession as a whole has resulted in large numbers of membership bodies each exercising overlapping regulatory functions and each jealously guarding its right to do so. Whereas the General Medical Council alone regulates the medical practitioner, there are, as of November 2020, ten PSA accredited organizations in respect of therapists, resulting in a cornucopia of acronyms: BACP, BPC, COSCA, AHPP, UKCP, ACP, ACC and others. Counsellors, as distinct from therapists,[4] may also be members of BAPT and PTUK.[5] Worse, the rules governing their disciplinary procedures vary significantly, but as will be seen, to no real purpose.

We have elected to concentrate upon four such bodies or regulators as illustrative of the sector: the Association of Child Psychotherapists (ACP), the British Association for Counselling & Psychotherapy (BACP), the British Psychoanalytic Council (BPC) and the UK Council for Psychotherapy (UKCP). A broader comparison would be unwieldy.

The complaint

A key question for any disciplinary body is 'who may complain?' Is it limited to the aggrieved patient,[6] or is a complaint by a third party admissible?

ACP (2019, para 4.4) imposes no restriction. Anyone can complain, save the anonymous. BPC and UKCP have omitted to address the issue. However, BACP has devoted a whole section to it (BACP, 2018, para 1.4).[7] Similarly, there is no consistency as to limitation periods. BPC (2016, para 1.7) and ACP (2019, para 4.3) demand that a complaint is brought within five years, UKCP (2017, para 3.3)[8] and BACP (2018 para 1.7(a)) ordinarily a mere three.

What happens if a Registrant[9] has resigned, whether through retirement or otherwise, before the complaint is made? May it still be pursued? Not according to BPC (2016, para 1.4.2) or ACP (2019, para 4.1.2). UKCP does assume jurisdiction provided the practitioner had been on its register at the time the impugned conduct took place (UKCP, 2017, para 3.1.2). BACP ploughs its own furrow, declaring that complaints are admissible against a former member provided the member was registered on or after 20 September 2013 (BACP, 2018, para 1.6(a)(ii)).

Often of real concern to a practitioner is the question of confidentiality.

Is he[10] free to respond fully, where to do so is to reveal otherwise confidential matters pertaining to the complainant? BPC considers the question worth addressing.[11] UKCP, BACP and ACP do not.

As each of the four regulators promises to provide the complainant with all relevant documentation,[12] a related anxiety is whether this must necessarily include the entirety of the practitioner's response, the contents of which may cause psychological harm.[13] None of the four have granted themselves the power to redact in the interests of the health of the complainant, implying that the question has not been considered. In practice, we find that most will eventually agree redactions in such circumstances, albeit with reluctance.

Screening

Assuming the complainant has identified the apposite acronym and has lodged a timely complaint in respect of a practitioner over which that regulator continues to exercise jurisdiction, the case then moves to its next stage, known as 'screening'.[14] For the practitioner, this is an anxious and often lengthy period that may, at least in theory, result in the discontinuance of proceedings. UKCP defines it as follows:

> The screening process is concerned with deciding, in a transparent and professional manner,[15] whether there is a **realistic prospect** that UKCP will be able to establish that the Registrant **may not be suitable** to be on the UKCP register without any restrictions or conditions of practice. (UKCP, 2017, para 6.1.)

UKCP entrusts this procedure to a Case Manager, unless the latter 'feels unable to make this decision' in which case it must be referred to the Professional Conduct Committee.

Contrast UKCP's test with that of ACP. Once received of a complaint in writing, signed and accompanied by pro forma authorization for its disclosure to the practitioner, ACP's Screening Group will consider whether the information received:

> **indicates a breach** of the Code **amounting to professional misconduct** may have occurred and that an investigation is called for to establish the facts.... (ACP, 2019, para 4.8.)

These are two quite distinct formulations. An 'indication' of a breach of a Code is in no sense the same as an assessment of the therapist's suitability to continue in practice.

BACP deploys a two-stage preliminary inquiry. First, the Case Manager will consider whether the complaint meets the 'threshold test', defined as being where:

> the facts alleged and evidenced by the Complainant, could, if proved, amount to **a failure** by the Member **to meet professional standards** … and is not vexatious and/or frivolous … (BACP, 2018, para 2.4.)

Assuming this low hurdle is surmounted, the complaint can be referred to BACP's Investigation and Assessment Committee (IAC), who will decide whether the 'proceedings test' is met. This largely reproduces the threshold test, which begs the question whether there is any real purpose served by the iteration:

> The proceedings test is met if in the opinion of the IAC, the facts alleged would (if proven) amount to **a failure to meet professional standards** … and there is a realistic prospect that facts justifying a finding of such a failure will be proved … and that it is in the public interest... (BACP, 2018, para 3.2(d).)

If so satisfied, the IAC then must allot the complaint to the Disciplinary Proceedings Track or to the Practice Review Process, the difference being that the first has exclusive jurisdiction over an allegation of professional misconduct.

Meanwhile, BPC's Screening Committee will refer a complaint to a Hearing Panel if:

> there is a realistic prospect of the Registrant's alleged conduct being substantiated or the alleged facts being proved and there is a realistic prospect of those facts being found to impair the Registrant's fitness to practise; and …. **that it would not be in the public interest**, because of the seriousness of the allegations or for any other reason, **for the matter to be resolved other than by way of the Hearing Panel process**. (BPC, 2016, para 3.7.3.)

BCP therefore allies itself to the UKCP structure, but adds a further element, namely consideration of the public interest in *not* pursuing the allegation.[16]

This somewhat tortuous construction is revelatory of a certain approach common to all the regulators. BCP's focus is not solely upon a just resolution of the instant complaint but as much in how the public at large may perceive it. Consequently, where it might otherwise be appropriate to address a complaint informally, the practitioner may nonetheless find himself pursued to a disciplinary hearing because BCP believes the public so demands. This reflects a commonplace of regulation, namely that the regulator must at all times uphold public confidence[17] in itself.

On their face, these four regulators apply four discrete filters. UKCP is interested in the practitioner's continuing suitability. BPC chooses to address his current impairment. ACP focuses upon his past professional misconduct. And BACP concerns itself with a similarly historical failure to meet professional standards.

It may seem as though the first two regulators concentrate upon the present, asking whether their practitioner, as of today, is impaired, whilst the other two concentrate upon the past, seeking to determine whether yesterday's act did indeed amount to misconduct. Yet delving deeper into the latitude each affords to its screening committee, there is a near convergence of outcome, if not of language. For example, UKCP treats past misconduct as evidence that a Registrant's present suitability is 'called into question' (UKCP, 2017, paras 2.1 and 2.1.1). ACP defines professional misconduct as that which 'might cause serious damage to the standing of the profession of child psychotherapy',[18] a statement broad enough to include conduct proscribed by all the other bodies. BPC does not define impairment of fitness to practise, but deems professional misconduct to constitute it (BPC, 2016, para 1.8.1). BACP declares that 'professional standards' means the 'standards that should reasonably be expected ... having regard to the Ethical Framework and any other code or rules issued for the purpose of this Procedure'.[19] BACP then links this to its definition of professional misconduct, being 'a failure to meet professional standards that is of sufficient seriousness that a period of suspension of membership or withdrawal of membership ... may be warranted'.

In truth, for each of our regulators, the past determines the present. What appears as two distinct tests, impairment and misconduct, in practice meld into one.

Is the public interest really served by such a cacophony?

And this is only the end of the beginning.

The response

What of the practitioner? By this stage he has received a formal complaint. He is informed that a screening process will take place. May he respond? Must he respond? What happens if he doesn't?

- UKCP 'invites' a response within 21 days of receipt of the complaint.
- BPC imposes a 21-day limit.
- ACP advises that the practitioner 'will be given the opportunity to respond' either in writing or in person at a time to be determined by the Investigating Panel.
- BACP's Case Manager 'may request further information ... within any time limit specified by the Case Manager'.[20]

All these regulators will proceed should the practitioner remain silent. However, BACP goes further, warning in effect that a failure to engage may later lead to the drawing of an adverse inference:

> If the Member does not respond promptly, or at all, to a request for information ... without reasonable explanation, this may be taken into account by the IAC should the complaint be referred to it... (BACP, 2018, para 2.3(d))

Why would a practitioner not set out his defence, in detail, at the earliest time available to him to do so? A common reason is that his policy of insurance does not cover the provision of legal advice in these preliminary stages. Many a practitioner requires legal assistance simply to navigate the Byzantine disciplinary process to which he is subject. If, in addition, the complaint may lead to the imposition of sanctions, let alone an interim suspension order,[21] the practitioner would be foolish to engage without a lawyer.[22] The risk is compounded by recent changes to the costs rules in civil cases,[23] the result of which is that any adverse finding by a regulator will place the complainant in an unassailable position should she also pursue a claim for damages for personal injury. Armed with that finding, and a law firm willing to take the case on a no-win-no-fee basis, there are now no costs implications for a patient/complainant, even if the claim is lost.[24]

The investigation

Each of the disciplinary procedures we are examining is expressly linked to an investigation conducted by officers of the professional body. This is to be expected. Proceedings that may adversely affect the livelihood and well-being of a practitioner should not be lightly undertaken.

BPC, however, expresses this obligation in almost hesitant tones:

> Either the SC at the time of referring the matter to the HP, or at any time the FtPO[25] or the Presenting Officer, **may consider** that further information or material should be obtained … in which case that further material **should if possible be obtained** … (BPC, 2016, para 5.5)

BACP is more forthright. Its Investigation and Assessment Committee:

> …may request such further information or make such further investigations as it considers appropriate… (BACP, 2018, 3.2(a))

ACP says the same for its Panel:

> The members of the Investigating Panel shall take such steps to investigate either jointly or alone as in their discretion they consider appropriate… (ACP, 2019, para 6.2)

UKCP invests authority in its Case Manager:

> The Case Manager may conduct such investigations as he considers reasonable and necessary (UKCP, 2017, para 6.6).

Notwithstanding these exhortations, none of the regulators have the experience, the staff, the time, the resources or indeed the inclination to conduct anything that might objectively be termed an investigation. In most of the cases in which we have acted, the complainant has not even been asked to disclose all the relevant material supporting her complaint, the investigators being content to rely upon her selection. The consequence is that the full context of the complaint, unless provided by the practitioner in an early response, is rarely available at the time the decision is made to proceed to a disciplinary hearing.

The allegations

If not already incorporated as part of the screening process, the next step will be the formulation of specific allegations. ACP does this by reference to its Code of Professional Conduct and Ethics, declaring that:

> … failure to fulfil the obligations laid down in this Code …. can result in the commencement of an investigation, the final outcome of which may be suspension, withdrawal of registration or other sanctions (ACP, 2017, para 1.3).

The complaint is consequently drafted so as to allege specific breaches of the Code.

UKCP also presents its case by reference to its own Code (UKCP, 2019).

BPC entrusts the drafting of the allegations to its Presenting Officer (BPC, 2016, para 5.6(i)), who is not obliged to link them to BPC's Code of Ethics or its (separate) Ethical Guidelines, but in practice does so.

BACP's procedure follows on from its focus upon a 'proceedings test'. The IAC must draft 'formal' allegations reflecting the conduct, but distinguishing in the body of the allegation where it is said to amount to professional misconduct (BACP, 2018, para 3.2(g)).

Unsurprisingly, such variation in approach results in wildly differing expressions of the same type of alleged misbehaviour. This might not matter much, were it obvious to the practitioner (and his lawyer) exactly what it is that has to be proved before a promising career hits the buffers. However, it rarely is, as the following example[26] demonstrates:

A client had previously made a number of attempts at suicide, usually resulting in in-patient psychiatric treatment. Following in-session discussions, the therapist had provided his personal mobile phone number and email address so that his client might, in extremis, reach him out of hours, thereby reducing the risks consequent upon suicidal ideation. His client did indeed initiate contact, leading to some intense exchanges at times of crisis. However, the therapist discouraged texts and emails out of crisis. Years later, the client complained that his former therapist should not have provided such private and intimate means of communication.

UKCP translated this complaint as follows:

That you, whilst acting in the capacity of a registered UKCP psychotherapist … engaged in the following behaviour:

    (a) Confused the existing therapeutic relationship with Client A, by way of encouraging the use of texting and email contact between sessions with Client A. This constitutes a breach of code 1.5 of UKCP's Ethical Principles and Code of Professional Conduct.

Code 1.5 is in the following, pithy terms:

1.5 – Psychotherapists are required to carefully consider possible implications of entering into dual or multiple relationships and make every effort to avoid entering into relationships that risk confusing an existing relationship and may impact adversely on a client. For example, a dual or multiple relationship could be a social or commercial relationship between the psychotherapist and client, or a supervisory relationship which runs alongside the therapeutic one. When dual or multiple relationships are unavoidable, for example in small communities, psychotherapists take responsibility to clarify and manage boundaries and confidentiality of the therapeutic relationship.

Taken together, what does all this mean? Is the gravamen of the allegation that the practitioner failed to 'carefully consider possible implications of entering into dual or multiple relationships?' If so, is it a complete answer to demonstrate that the practitioner *did* so consider but concluded that since there was no dual relationship, there were no implications? Or is it sufficient to show that there was no real risk of confusion, regardless of whether the practitioner had given any thought to anything else? Or is it enough that objectively, the impugned act was unlikely to 'impact adversely on a client'? Or is the allegation proved where the Disciplinary Panel, exercising perfect hindsight, substitutes its own judgment for that of the practitioner?

The disciplinary panel

At some point every practitioner asks, 'Who shall judge me?' The unsatisfactory response he receives is, 'It depends'. The related question 'Who will know about it?' is also met with the same answer.

UKCP appoints an Adjudication Panel. This comprises three persons, two of whom must be therapists. The Chair will be a layperson. One of the therapists must be from the same modality as the Registrant (UKCP, 2017, paras 7.2 and 7.3).

BACP prefers a Professional Conduct Panel. This must be not less than three persons, including one lay person and at least one member of BACP (i.e. a therapist). There is no requirement for that member to share the modality of the practitioner. The Chair is appointed by the Registrar (BACP, 2018, para 4.1(b) and (c)).

BPC deploys a Hearing Panel. This too has three persons, one of whom is lay and another, a current or former BPC registrant, who need not be of the modality of the practitioner. The Chair is appointed by the Complaints Management Committee (BPC, 2016, para 5.1).

ACP has a Disciplinary Panel. Its three members are taken from ACP's Ethical Practice Group and 'so far as practicable' should consist of those whose experience or expertise 'may be material to the issues in question'. Additionally, 'unless it is wholly impracticable' the Disciplinary Panel 'will have a majority of lay members'[27]. In an unusually serious or complex case, a member of the Legal Members Panel may also be appointed. The Chair of the Disciplinary Panel is appointed by the Chair of the Ethical Practice Group (ACP, 2019, para 8.1).

Public or private?

- ACP's Disciplinary Panel sits in private (ACP, 2019, para 8.14).
- BPC's Hearing Panel sits in private (BPC, 2016, para 5.19).
- UKCP's Adjudication Panel sits in public but exceptionally may sit in private on a case-by-case basis (UKCP, 2017, para 7.8).
- Conversely, BACP's Professional Conduct Panel sits in private but may sit in public when the Panel considers that a private hearing would be contrary to the public interest (BACP, 2018, para 5.2(b) and (c)).

Rules of evidence and procedure

What constitutes admissible evidence is a core consideration for the parties to any formal hearing in any jurisdiction. It will perhaps by now come as little surprise that each of the four regulators takes a different course, although there is some commonality. All apply the civil standard of proof, as now deployed by all statutory regulators across all regulatory sectors. Each imposes upon its Presenting Officer[28] the burden of proving the case to that standard. However, the differences are marked.

BPC's approach is the most prescriptive and clearly culled from both the civil and criminal procedure rules. Each party must serve in writing all the evidence upon which it intends to rely at least 28 days before the hearing. Witness statements must be signed and dated. Either party may request the other to ensure the attendance of their witness, although the Hearing Panel has a discretion to admit the statement in the absence of the witness. Objections to the admissibility of documentary evidence must be notified at least 21 days in advance. A witness's statement stands as her evidence in chief, although supplementary questions may be asked. A Registrant acting in person may not cross-examine a complainant in a case involving a sexual allegation. The Hearing Panel may order measures[29] including video links, screens and pre-recorded evidence to maximize the quality of a witness's evidence.[30]

UKCP allows its Adjudication Panel to admit any evidence if it is 'relevant to the case and its admission is fair to the parties' (UKCP, 2017, para 7.14). The parties must provide the secretary to the Panel and each other all the documents including witness statements upon which they rely at least 28 days in advance. Vulnerable witnesses may receive special measures.

ACP asserts that its own procedures shall be subject to 'the overriding objective ... to deal justly with the case before it ... at any stage at which the Disciplinary Panel is to exercise its discretion, it shall do so with regard to the overriding objective' (ACP, 2019, para 9.1).[31] The discretion afforded to the Panel is substantial, because ACP also declares that 'the rules of evidence do not apply at the hearing' (ACP, 2019, para 9.8).

BACP also dispenses with rules of evidence (BACP, 2018, para 4.9(a)). Lest there be lingering doubt, BACP further enjoins the Panel to 'admit oral, documentary or other evidence, whether or not such evidence would be admissible in civil or criminal proceedings, subject to any relevant statutory requirements and the requirements of relevance and fairness' (BACP, 2018, para 4.9(b)). The Panel is also the master of its own procedure, which expressly includes the power to make orders for special measures (BACP, 2018, paras 4.5 and 5.6(j)–(l)).

Who prosecutes?[32]

This question divides into two, namely who conducts the case against the practitioner and on whose behalf does he do so?

BPC's FtPO[33] appoints an independent lawyer to act as Presenting Officer (BPC, 2016, para 5.5). Although not specifically addressed, the Complaints Procedure is predicated upon the Presenting Officer acting on behalf of BPC itself.

ACP instructs members of its Investigating Panel to present the case, who are then treated as one of the two parties to the Disciplinary Hearing (ACP, 2019, para 6.1). By so doing, ACP makes itself the prosecutor.

BACP declares that the parties to a complaint 'are the Association and the Member' and that the complaint 'will be presented by the Association'. The Registrar appoints a Case Presenter (BACP, 2018, para 4.2).[34]

UKCP's Case Manager may act as Presenting Officer, or he may instruct an independent lawyer to do so. UKCP is also unambiguous as to its role. Before an Adjudication Panel the parties are UKCP on the one hand, and the Registrant on the other. The Complainant, lest there be doubt, has the status of witness (UKCP, 2017, para 7.1).

All four regulators would describe their own procedures as reflecting contemporary standards of fairness. Were this not so, they would surely not be accredited. BACP goes further still, insisting that its own Case Presenter 'be fair and objective' (BACP, 2018, para 4.3(a)).

Yet in practice, and especially from the perspective of the practitioner, the conduct of the regulator as prosecutor rarely seems anything other than partisan. The reasons for this have already been touched upon. The absence of an investigation will usually leave the Presenting Officer relying entirely upon the complainant to prove his case, thus prompting him to challenge the veracity of contradictory or undermining evidence. The practitioner's sense of disquiet is compounded when the Presenting Officer further relies upon documentary evidence that has been selectively chosen by the complainant alone.

As we have seen, the language of objectivity is plentifully deployed by all four professional bodies. However, the structure of each belies the rhetoric. Stripped down, the regulator is the prosecutor. And the prosecutor sets the rules and appoints the judges.

It need not be like this.

One code

Whatever the educational and other merits of the existing professional bodies, there is no public interest in permitting each to exercise its own version of a disciplinary code. There should be one code, contained within one document, and expressed in tightly worded but comprehensible language. It should contain all procedural and evidential rules. At its heart should be the concept of 'misconduct'.[35]

Misconduct: a simple test

We suggest that all impugned acts can and should be drafted in terms of 'misconduct'. As we have sought to demonstrate, the impairment test is itself a disguised test of misconduct. That is not to deny it all value. Impairment will always be a critical factor when considering the appropriate sanction, if any. But it should have no part to play in determining the quality of the impugned act.

What is misconduct? Misconduct arises, and only arises, when a practitioner's conduct falls 'far below the standard of the reasonably competent practitioner'. Misconduct is therefore proved where (a) the disciplinary panel is satisfied that the impugned act took place, and (b) that act fell far below the requisite standard. The first of these is a question of fact. The second is a question of judgment. Cases on the margin may require expert evidence as to what constitutes the contemporary standard, but we doubt that there will be many. Most will turn upon the answer to the first question.

Conduct falling short of misconduct

Conduct that does not meet the test of misconduct but nonetheless falls below[36] the requisite standard should be presumed capable of remediation through supervision. A supervisor's report may be ordered. Repetition of the conduct will ordinarily amount to misconduct.

Cases where others should investigate first

Where the police or other criminal enforcement agencies are already involved (in cases of serious sexual misconduct for example) a judgment will need to be made about whether to await the outcome of the police enquiry or to run a parallel investigation. A primary consideration is whether to do so might prejudice the criminal case.[37] An interim suspension order may often be appropriate.

Publicity

A finding of misconduct should be published only when it is in the public interest to do so. Conduct that is capable of remediation, whether or not it also amounts to misconduct, would rarely, we suggest, meet the public interest test.

Screening

The purpose of screening is to ensure that the practitioner is protected from manifestly unfounded or vexatious complaints. If a single test of misconduct were adopted, this should become a relatively straightforward exercise.

Investigation and disclosure

The current system of investigation over-promises and under-delivers. The smaller professional bodies cannot afford the cost of investigation. The very largest might, but doesn't. There is no justification for a continuation of the related and commonplace practice of relying upon the complainant to select the relevant documents to support the case against the practitioner. At the very least, the task of a responsible investigating officer should be to act as a filter, ensuring that only those aspects of the complainant's narrative that are objectively capable of amounting to misconduct are referred onwards for adjudication. The investigating officer, not the complainant, should decide which documents are advanced in support of any pleaded allegation. Documents not so used should ordinarily be made available to the practitioner, unless wholly irrelevant.

The professional disciplinary centre

In the absence of a statutory scheme, the many failings we have identified might be addressed if the various regulators are willing to co-operate.

We propose that the professional bodies merge their disciplinary functions through the creation of a Disciplinary Centre that would have sole responsibility for the entire disciplinary process, including appeal.[38] Given adequate funding, we envisage that such an entity would over time engender that which is so sorely lacking today, namely the confidence and trust of complainant, practitioner and citizen alike.

Notes

1. For these purposes 'therapist' means a practitioner who is not subject to a statutory scheme of regulation.
2. The various appellate procedures together with the supervision of the High Court do bring the proceedings to an end – eventually, but at considerable cost.
3. Those that do not are either squeezed out by market forces or unable to obtain professional indemnity insurance or both – or so it is said. We know of no research that establishes this. We doubt the charlatan or the wide-eyed enthusiast would be deterred by lack of insurance.
4. The terms are usually treated as synonymous, but not on the PSA website.
5. The absence of full titles is deliberate, as the bewilderment generated may mirror that of a prospective patient or interested observer.
6. Our use of 'patient' should be understood to include 'client'. Some regulators prefer the former, others the latter.
7. BACP (2018), para 1.4: essentially the patient or authorized representative, legal guardian and BACP itself.
8. UKCP (2017), para 3.3. The case manager has a discretion to waive the limitation.
9. A 'Registrant' is a practitioner who has been admitted to the register of a

professional body. The term is used by most professional bodies but not all. ACP and BACP prefer 'Member'. We prefer 'practitioner'.

10. As 'he/she' is clumsy and 'they' too modern, 'she' and 'he' are to be understood as interchangeable here and hereafter.

11. BPC (2016), para 2.4. '...the Registrant is released from the obligation of confidentiality ... to the extent reasonably required to ... respond'.

12. BACP (2018), para 3.3(d); BPC (2016), para 3.5; ACP (2019), para 6.4; UKCP (2017), para 6.3.

13. For example, supervision notes where the complainant is discussed in impersonal and theoretical terms that are apt to be misconstrued.

14. But not by BACP, which prefers 'Preliminary Investigation'.

15. A curiously redundant and therefore revealing statement.

16. BACP imposes a similar condition upon its IAC, but expressed positively.

17. The terms 'public interest' or 'confidence' are nowhere defined. In practice public interest and prurient interest seem indistinguishable.

18. ACP (2017), para 7.1. Interestingly, two of the four examples provided concern the interrelationship of ACP members, which perhaps tells its own story.

19. BACP (2018) 'Definitions'.

20. UKCP (2017), para 6.3; BPC (2016), para 3.5; ACP (2019), para 6.3; BACP (2018), para 2.3(d).

21. All the regulators have granted themselves the power to make interim orders, including suspension.

22. Yes, we would say that. It is true nonetheless.

23. QOCS, that is, qualified one-way costs shifting. In a claim for personal injury, the civil court cannot now award the successful defendant his costs unless he can show that the claim made against him was fraudulent. Where a regulator has found misconduct, it will only be in the most exceptional circumstances that the practitioner will be able to surmount that hurdle.

24. Which is unlikely. Given the costs risks, the practitioner will probably find that his insurance company chooses to settle the claim, regardless of the merits.

25. All these abbreviations are in the original.

26. From a real case, anonymized. There were a number of allegations of a similar type. This was one.

27. As of April 2018, ACP's Ethical Practice Group must contain at least six lay members and no more than eight.

28. That is, the equivalent of prosecuting counsel in a criminal court.

29. In the criminal courts these are collectively known as 'special measures', a term we adopt.

30. These are but some of the provisions: see BPC (2016) paras 5.6–5.17.

31. This is lifted directly from the corresponding provision in the Criminal Procedure Rules.

32. 'Prosecutes' in this context means 'conduct the proceedings'. Most professional bodies prefer the anodyne 'presenting officer'.

33. We relent. Fitness to Practise Officer.
34. The Case Presenter need not be a lawyer in independent practice, but often is.
35. The scheme may also provide for a small set of other defined categories where the regulator can take action, for example, findings of another (relevant) regulator, convictions, and so on.
36. But not far below.
37. By way of example, a coroner's inquest will be adjourned pending the conclusion of extant criminal proceedings.
38. The High Court should retain its supervisory jurisdiction, but limited to review, not appeal.

REFERENCES

Chapter 1

Middleton, W. (2013). 'Parent-child incest that extends into adulthood: a survey of international press reports, 2007–2011'. *Journal of Trauma and Dissociation*, 14, 184–197.

Middleton, W., Sachs, A. and Dorahy, M. (eds) (2018). *The Abused and the Abuser: Victim-Perpetrator Dynamics*. London, New York: Routledge.

Nedergaard-Couchman, R. and Attavar, R. (2022). 'Complaints and incident procedures for NHS clinicians'. In A. Sachs and V. Sinason (eds), *The Psychotherapist and the Professional Complaint: The Shadow Side of Therapy*. London: Karnac Books.

Sachs, A. (2007). 'Infanticidal attachment: symbolic and concrete'. *Attachment: New Directions in Psychotherapy and Relational Psychoanalysis*, 1(3), 297–304.

Sachs, A. (2011). 'As thick as thieves, or the ritual abuse family: an attachment perspective on a forensic relationship'. In V. Sinason (ed.), *Attachment, Trauma and Multiplicity*. 2nd edn, Hove: Brunner-Routledge.

Sachs, A. (2013) 'Still being hurt: the vicious cycle of dissociative disorders, attachment and ongoing abuse'. *Attachment: New Directions in Psychotherapy and Relational Psychoanalysis*, 7(1), 90–100.

Sachs, A. (2017) 'Through the lens of attachment relationship: stable DID, active DID and other trauma-based mental disorders'. *Journal of Trauma & Dissociation*, 18(3), 319–339.

Salter, M. (2013). *Organised Sexual Abuse*. Abingdon: Routledge.

Sinason, V. (2011) *Attachment, Trauma and Multiplicity*. 2nd edn, New York: Routledge.

Sinason, V. (2022). 'Complaints in the field of dissociative disorders: six key categories'. In A. Sachs and V. Sinason (eds), *The Psychotherapist and the Professional Complaint: The Shadow Side of Therapy*. London: Karnac Books.

Winnicott, D. (1949). 'Hate in the counter-transference'. *International Journal of Psycho-Analysis*, 30, 69–74.

Winnicott, D. (1973). *The Child, the Family, and the Outside World* (pp. 115–116). Penguin.

Chapter 2

Bleger, J. (1967). 'Psycho-analysis of the psychoanalytic frame'. *The International Journal of Psychoanalysis*, 48(4), 511–519.

Bordin, E. S. (1979). 'The generalizability of the psychoanalytic concept of the working alliance'. *Psychotherapy: Theory, Research & Practice* 16 (3): 252–60.

Clarkson, P. (1993). 'On psychotherapy'. Whurr Publishers Ltd, England.

Cozolino, L. (2006). 'The neuroscience of human relationships' W.W. Norton, New York.

DeYoung, P. A. (2015). 'Understanding and treating chronic shame a/neurobiological approach' Routledge, New York.

Farber & Doolin (2011). 'Positive Regard'. *Journal of Society for the Advancement of Psychotherapy* 48: 58–64.

Frank, J.D. (1979). 'The present status of outcome studies'. *Journal of Consulting and Clinical Psychology* 47(1) 310–16.

Gelso, C. J. (2019). 'The therapeutic relationship in psychotherapy practice' Routledge, Oxford.

Klein, M. (1997). 'Envy and Gratitude and Other Works 1946–1963'. Vintage, London.

Kolden, Klein, Wang, & Austin (2011). 'Congruence/genuineness'. *Journal of the American Psychological Association* 48 (1), 65–71.

Mackewn, J. (1997). 'Developing Gestalt Counselling' Sage Publications, London.

May, R. (1969) 'Love and Will', W.W. Norton, New York.

Chapter 3

Bentham, J. (1995). *The Panopticon Writings*. M. Bozovic (ed), London and New York: Verso.

Berman, E. (1993). 'Psychoanalysis, rescue and utopia'. *Utopian Studies*, 4(2), 44–56.

Foucault, M. (2011). *Courage of the Truth (the Government of Self and Others II): Lectures at the Collège de France, 1983–1984*. London: Palgrave-Macmillan.

Freud, S. (1957) 'A special type of choice of object made by men'. In *The Standard Edition of the Complete Psychological Works of Sigmund Freud Vol. 11* (pp. 163–176). London: Hogarth, 1957.

Heinonen, E. and Nissen-Lie, H. A. (2019) 'The professional and personal characteristics of effective psychotherapists: a systematic review'. *Psychotherapy Research*, 30(4), 1–16.

Herman, J. (1992). *Trauma and Recovery*. New York: Basic Books.

Juvenal (1992). *The Satires*. N. Rudd (trans.). Oxford: Oxford University Press.

Kearns, A (2006) 'Professional Development and Informed Practise in the Area of Ethical Complaints.' Middlesex University/Metanoia Institute.

Kearns, A. (2007/2011). *The Mirror Crack'd: When Good Enough Therapy Goes Wrong and Other Cautionary Tales for the Humanistic Practitioner*. London: Karnac Books.

Lambert, M. J. (1986). 'Implications of psychotherapy outcome research for eclectic psychotherapy'. In J. C. Norcross (ed.), *Handbook of eclectic psychotherapy* (pp. 436–462). New York: Brunner/Mazel.

Lambert, M. J., and Barley, D. E. (2001). 'Research summary on the therapeutic relationship and psychotherapy outcome'. *Psychotherapy: Theory, Research, Practice, Training*, 38(4), 357–361.

UK Council for Psychotherapy (UKCP). Annual review of accreditation 2019/20. November 2019

Chapter 4

Cook, B. (2014) Restorative justice can drastically reduce need to restrain young offenders. *The Guardian* www.theguardian.com/social-care-network/2014/feb/04/restorative-justice-reduce-restrain-young-offenders (accessed 4 July 2022).

Herman, J. L. (1992). *Trauma and Recovery: From Domestic Abuse to Political Terror*. Rivers Oram Press/Pandora List.

Munro, E. and Turnell, A. (2018). 'Re-designing organizations to facilitate rights-based practice in child protection. In A. Falch-Erikson and E. Backe-Hanson (eds), *Human Rights in Child Protection*. Palgrave Macmillan.

NHS Resolution (2019). *Being Fair: Supporting a just and learning culture for staff and patients following incidents in the NHS*. https://resolution.nhs.uk/resources/being-fair/.

Victim Support (2010). *Victims' Justice? What victims and witnesses really want from sentencing*.

Chapter 5

Badouk Epstein, O., Schwartz, J. and Wingfield Schwartz, R. (2011). *Ritual Abuse and Mind Control: The Manipulation of Attachment Needs*. London: Routledge.

Bowman, C. G., and Mertz, E. (1996). 'A dangerous direction: legal intervention in sexual abuse survivor therapy'. *Harvard Law Review*, 109(3), 549–639. https://doi.org/10.2307/1342066

De Mause, L. (1974). *The History of Childhood*. New York: Harper and Row.

Fonagy, P. and Target. M. (1995). 'Dissociation and trauma'. *Current Opinions in Psychiatry*, 8, 161–166.

Gabbard, G. O. (ed) (1989). *Sexual Exploitation in Professional Relationships*. American Psychiatric Press.

Johns, J. (2022). 'What if I should die?'. In V. Sinason and A. Conway (eds), *Trauma and Memory: The Science and the Silenced*, Abingdon: Routledge.

Kahr, B. (2007). 'The infanticidal attachment'. *Attachment: New Directions in Psychotherapy and Relational Psychoanalysis*, 1(2) 117–232.

Liotti, G. (1992). 'Disorganised disorientated attachment in the etiology of the dissociative disorders'. *Dissociation*, 5, 196–204.

Orr, M. (1996). 'Culture of Fear'. *Counselling News*, March 1996.

Pope, K. and Vetter, V. A. (1991). 'Prior therapist-patient sexual involvement among patients seen by psychologists'. *Psychotherapy; Theory, Research, Practice, Training*, 28(3), 429–38.

Pope, K. S., Vasquez, M. J. T., Chavez-Duenas, N. Y. and Adames, H. Y. (2021). 'Sexual attraction to patients, therapist vulnerabilities, and sexual relationships with patients'. In *Ethics in Psychotherapy and Counseling: A Practical Guide* (pp. 327–356). Hoboken NJ: Wiley.

Sachs, A. (2008). 'Infanticidal attachment: the link between dissociative identity disorder and crime'. In A. Sachs and G. Galton (eds), *Forensic Aspects of Dissociative Identity Disorder* (pp. 127–139). London: Taylor and Francis.

Sachs, A. (2011). 'As thick as thieves, or the ritual abuse family: an attachment perspective on a forensic relationship'. In Sinason, V. (ed.) *Attachment, Trauma and Multiplicity*. 2nd edn, (pp. 75–82). Hove: Brunner-Routledge.

Sachs, A. (2013). 'Still being hurt: the vicious cycle of dissociative disorders, attachment and ongoing abuse'. *Attachment: New Directions in Psychotherapy and Relational Psychoanalysis*, 7(1), 90–100.

Sachs, A. (2017). 'Through the lens of attachment relationship: stable DID, active DID and other trauma-based mental disorders'. *Journal of Trauma & Dissociation*, 18(3), 319–339.

Sachs, A. and Galton, G. (eds) (2008). *Forensic Aspects of Dissociative Identity Disorder*. London: Taylor & Francis.

Sinason, V. (1990). 'Passionate lethal attachments'. *British Journal of Psychotherapy*, 7(1).

Sinason, V. (1992). *Mental Handicap and the Human Condition: New Approaches from the Tavistock*. London: Free Association Books.

Sinason, V. (2017). 'Dying for love: an attachment problem with some perpetrator introjects'. *Journal of Trauma & Dissociation*, 18(3), 340–355.

Sinason, V. (2020). *The Truth about Trauma and Dissociation: Everything You Didn't Want to Know and Were Afraid to Ask*. London: Confer Books.

Sinason, V. (2022). *The Orpheus Project*. London: Sphinx Books.

Chapter 6

Anonymous (1948). 'Profile: The American Psychoanalytic Association'. *Bulletin of the American Psychoanalytic Association*, 4(1), 5–10.

Anonymous (1981). 'Changes in Membership'. *Bulletin of the American Psychoanalytic Association*, 37(1), 469–471. In *Journal of the American Psychoanalytic Association*, 29, 469–485.

Baddeley, A. (1982). *Your Memory: A User's Guide*. London: Sidgwick and Jackson/ Multimedia Publications (UK).

Baddeley, A. (2004). *Your Memory: A User's Guide. New Illustrated Edition*. London: Carlton Books.

Bos, J. and Groenendijk, L. (2007). 'Marginalization Through Psychoanalysis: An Introduction'. In J. Bos and L. Groenendijk, *The Self-Marginalization of Wilhelm Stekel: Freudian Circles Inside and Out* (pp. 1–16). New York: Springer/Springer Science and Business Media.

Clark-Lowes, F. (2010). *Freud's Apostle: Wilhelm Stekel and the Early History of Psychoanalysis*. Gamlingay, Sandy, Bedfordshire: Authors on Line.

Deutsch, H. (1973). *Confrontations with Myself: An Epilogue*. New York: W.W. Norton and Company.

Farrell, E. (2006). 'The Presence of the Body in Psychotherapy'. In G. Galton (ed.), *Touch Papers: Dialogues on Touch in the Psychoanalytic Space* (pp. 97–108). London: Karnac Books.

Freeman, L. (1992). *Why Norma Jean Killed Marilyn Monroe*. Chicago, Illinois: Global Rights.

Freud, S. (1896). 'L'Hérédité et l'étiologie des névroses'. *Revue Neurologique*, 4, 161–169.

Freud, S. (1910a). Letter to Sándor Ferenczi, 13th February. In E. Brabant, E. Falzeder, P. Giampieri-Deutsch, and A. Haynal (eds.) (1993) *Sigmund Freud and Sándor Ferenczi, Briefwechsel: Band I/1 1908–1911* (pp. 212–214). Vienna: Böhlau Verlag/Böhlau Verlag Gesellschaft.

Freud, S. (1910b). Letter to Sándor Ferenczi, 13th February. In E. Brabant, E. Falzeder, P. Giampieri-Deutsch, and A. Haynal (eds.), P. T. Hoffer (trans.), (1993), *The Correspondence of Sigmund Freud and Sándor Ferenczi: Volume I, 1908–1914* (pp. 136–138). Cambridge, Massachusetts: Belknap Press of Harvard University Press.

Freud, S. (1914). Letter to Ernest Jones, 21st February. In R. A. Paskauskas (ed.) (1993), *The Complete Correspondence of Sigmund Freud and Ernest Jones: 1908–1939*, F. Voss (trans.), (p. 264). Cambridge, Massachusetts: Belknap Press of Harvard University Press.

Freud, S. (1918). 'Aus der Geschichte einer infantilen Neurose'. In *Sammlung kleiner Schriften zur Neurosenlehre: Vierte Folge* (pp. 578–717). Vienna: Hugo Heller und Compagnie.

Freud, S. (1923a). Letter to Fritz Wittels, 18th December. In E. L. Freud (ed.) (1960), *Briefe: 1873–1939* (pp. 345–346). Frankfurt am Main: S. Fischer Verlag.

Freud, S. (1923b). Letter to Fritz Wittels, 18th December. In E. L. Freud (ed.) (1960), *Letters of Sigmund Freud*, T. Stern and J. Stern (trans.), (pp. 345–347). New York: Basic Books.

Freud, S. (1924a). Letter to Fritz Wittels, 15th August. In E. L. Freud (ed.) (1960), *Briefe: 1873–1939* (pp. 350–353). Frankfurt am Main: S. Fischer Verlag.

Freud, S. (1924b). Letter to Karl Abraham, 28th November. In S. Freud and K. Abraham (2009), *Briefwechsel 1907–1925: Vollständige Ausgabe. Band 2: 1915–1925*, E. Falzeder and L. M. Hermanns (eds.) (pp. 791–793). Vienna: Verlag Turia und Kant.

Freud, S. and Freud, A. (1924). Circular Letter Number 1, 15th December. In K. Abraham (2002), *The Complete Correspondence of Sigmund Freud and Karl Abraham: 1907–1925. Completed Edition*, E. Falzeder (ed.) C. Schwarzacher, C. Trollope and K. Majthényi King (trans.) (pp. 528–529). London: H. Karnac (Books).

Geib, P. (1998). 'The Experience of Nonerotic Physical Contact in Traditional Psychotherapy'. In E. W. L. Smith, P. R. Clance and S. Imes (eds.), *Touch in Psychotherapy: Theory, Research, and Practice* (pp. 109–126). New York: Guilford Press.

Greenson, R. R. (1978a). *Explorations in Psychoanalysis*. New York: International Universities Press.

Greenson, R. R. (1978b). 'Special Problems in Psychotherapy with the Rich and Famous.' Box 2, Folder 19. Ralph R. Greenson Collection, Department of Special Collections, University of California at Los Angeles, Los Angeles, California, USA. Cited in Donald Spoto (1993). *Marilyn Monroe: The Biography*, p. 649, n. 427. New York: HarperCollins Publishers.

Grinker, R., Snr (1985). 'A Memoir of My Psychoanalytic Education'. J. Martin (ed.), *Psychoanalytic Education*, 4, 3–12.

James, O. (1997). Personal Communication to the Author. 24th May.

Jones, E. (1955). *The Life and Work of Sigmund Freud: Volume 2. Years of Maturity. 1901–1919*. New York: Basic Books.

Jones, E. (1957). *The Life and Work of Sigmund Freud: Volume 3.The Last Phase. 1919–1939*. New York: Basic Books.

Kahr, B. (1999). Book Review of P. Roazen. *How Freud Worked: First-Hand Accounts of Patients. Psychoanalysis and History*, 1, 273–281.

Kahr, B. (2004). 'Juvenile Paedophilia: The Psychodynamics of an Adolescent'. In C. W. Socarides and L. R. Loeb (eds.), *The Mind of the Paedophile: Psychoanalytic Perspectives* (pp. 95–119). London: H. Karnac (Books).

Kahr, B. (2020). *Bombs in the Consulting Room: Surviving Psychological Shrapnel*. London and Abingdon, Oxfordshire: Routledge/Taylor & Francis Group.

Kahr, B. (2021). *Freud's Pandemics: Surviving Global War, Spanish Flu, and the Nazis*. London: Karnac Books.

Kahr, B. (2022). 'Freud's Blurry Boundaries: Unconscious Transmission of Technique Across the Ages'. In A. Sachs and V. Sinason (eds.), *Out of Hours: Boundary Adjustment*. London and Abingdon: Routledge [In press].

Kirsner, D. (2000). *Unfree Associations: Inside Psychoanalytic Institutes*. London: Process Press.

MacLean, G. and Rappen, U. (1991). *Hermine Hug-Hellmuth: Her Life and Work*. New York: Routledge/Routledge, Chapman and Hall.

Miller, J. J. (2014). *Marilyn Monroe & Joe DiMaggio: Love in Japan, Korea & Beyond*. New Jersey: J. J. Avenue Productions.

Reich, W. (1927). *Die Funktion des Orgasmus: Zur Psychopathologie und zur Soziologie des Geschlechtslebens*. Vienna: Internationaler Psychoanalytischer Verlag.

Reich, W. (1942). *The Discovery of the Orgone: Volume One The Function of the Orgasm: Sex-Economic Problems of Biological Energy*. T. P. Wolfe (trans.). New York: Orgone Institute Press.

Reich, W. (1948). Personal Communication to Myron Sharaf. Quoted in Myron Sharaf (1983), *Fury on Earth: A Biography of Wilhelm Reich* (p. 117). New York: St. Martin's Press/Marek.

Roazen, P. (1969). *Brother Animal: The Story of Freud and Tausk*. New York: Alfred A. Knopf.

Roazen, P. (1975). *Freud and His Followers*. New York: Alfred A. Knopf.

Roazen, P. (1985). *Helene Deutsch: A Psychoanalyst's Life*. Garden City, New York: Anchor Press/Doubleday.

Roazen, P. (1995). *How Freud Worked: First-Hand Accounts of Patients*. Northvale, New Jersey: Jason Aronson.

Roazen, P. (2005). *Edoardo Weiss: The House That Freud Built*. New Brunswick, New Jersey: Transaction Publishers.

Sharaf, M. (1971a). Interview with Grete Bibring, 10th April. Cited in M. Sharaf (1983), *Fury on Earth: A Biography of Wilhelm Reich* (p. 490, n. 7). New York: St. Martin's Press/Marek.

Sharaf, M. (1971b). Interview with Grete Bibring, 30th May. Cited in M. Sharaf (1983), *Fury on Earth: A Biography of Wilhelm Reich* (p. 491, n. 20). New York: St. Martin's Press/Marek.

Sharaf, M. (1971c). Interview with Lia Laszky, 15th July. Cited in M. Sharaf (1983), *Fury on Earth: A Biography of Wilhelm Reich* (p. 493, n. 4). New York: St. Martin's Press/Marek.

Sharaf, M. (1971d). Interview with Gladys Meyer, 16th July. Cited in M. Sharaf (1983). *Fury on Earth: A Biography of Wilhelm Reich* (p. 515, n. 6). New York: St. Martin's Press/Marek.

Sharaf, M. (1972). Interview with Ola Raknes, 5th July. Cited in M. Sharaf (1983). *Fury on Earth: A Biography of Wilhelm Reich* (p. 504, n. 2). New York: St. Martin's Press/Marek.

Sharaf, M. (1983). *Fury on Earth: A Biography of Wilhelm Reich*. New York: St. Martin's Press/Marek.

Smith, E. W. L. (1998a). 'Traditions of Touch in Psychotherapy'. In E. W. L. Smith, P. R. Clance and S. Imes (eds.), *Touch in Psychotherapy: Theory, Research, and Practice* (pp. 3–15). New York: Guilford Press, Guilford Publications.

Smith, E. W. L. (1998b). 'A Taxonomy and Ethics of Touch in Psychotherapy'. In E. W. L. Smith, P. R. Clance and S. Imes (eds.), *Touch in Psychotherapy: Theory, Research, and Practice* (pp. 36–51). New York: Guilford Press, Guilford Publications.

Spoto, D. (1993). *Marilyn Monroe: The Biography*. New York: HarperCollins Publishers.

Stanton, M. (1988). Personal Communication to the Author, 14th January.

Stekel, W. (1909). 'Beiträge zur Traumdeutung'. *Jahrbuch für psychoanalytische und psychopathologische Forschungen*, 1, 458–512.

Stekel, W. (1910). 'Warum sie den eigenen Namen hassen'. *Zentralblatt für Psychoanalyse*, 1, 109.

Stekel, W. (1911). *Die Sprache des Traumes: Eine Darstellung der Symbolik und Deutung des Traumes in ihren Beziehungen zur kranken und gesunden Seele für Ärzte und Psychologen*. Wiesbaden: J. F. Bergmann.

Stekel, W. (1926). 'Zur Geschichte der analytischen Bewegung'. *Fortschritte der Sexualwissenschaft und Psychanalyse*, 2, 539–575.

Stekel, W. (1948). 'Autobiography (V)'. *American Journal of Psychotherapy*, 2, 256–282.

Stekel, W. (1950). *The Autobiography of Wilhelm Stekel: The Life Story of a Pioneer Psychoanalyst*. E. A. Gutheil (ed.), New York: Liveright Publishing Corporation.

Sterba, R. F. (1982). *Reminiscences of a Viennese Psychoanalyst*. Detroit, Michigan: Wayne State University Press.

Totton, N. (2020). *Body Psychotherapy for the 21st Century*. London: Confer/Confer Books.

Training Committee Minutes: .Training Ctte Minutes: 24.3.1926–29.10.1945. Archives of the British Psychoanalytical Society, British Psychoanalytical Society, Byron House, Maida Vale, London.

Walker, E. and Young, P. D. (1986). *A Killing Cure*. New York: Henry Holt and Company.

Winnicott, D. W. (1949). 'Hate in the Counter-Transference'. *International Journal of Psycho-Analysis*, 30, 69–74.

Wittels, F. (1992). 'Reconciliation with Freud'. In E. Timms and R. Robertson (eds.), *Psychoanalysis in its Cultural Context: Austrian Studies III* (pp. 57–70). Edinburgh: Edinburgh University Press.

Wittels, F. (1995). *Freud and the Child Woman: The Memoirs of Fritz Wittels*. E. Timms (ed.), New Haven, Connecticut: Yale University Press.

Chapter 7

Adshead, G. (1994). 'Looking for clues: a review of the literature on false allegations of sexual abuse'. In V. Sinason (ed.), *Treating Survivors of Satanist Abuse*. London: Routledge.

Bentovim, A. (1992). *Trauma-Organized Systems: Physical and Sexual Abuse in Families*. London: Karnac Books.

Bion, W. R. (1959). 'Attacks on linking'. *International Journal of Psycho-analysis*, 40.

Bion, W. R. (1962b). 'A theory of thinking'. *International Journal of Psycho-analysis*, 53.

Bion, W. R. (1967). *Second Thoughts*. London: Heinemann.

Bion, W. R. (1990). *Brazilian Lectures*. Karnac Books.

Boston, M. and Lush, D. (1994). 'Further considerations of methodology for evaluating psychoanalytic psychotherapy with children'. *Journal of Child Psychotherapy*, 20(2), 205–229.

Boston, M. and Szur, R. (1983). *Psychotherapy with Severely Deprived Children*. London: Routledge.

Freud, S. (1915a). 'Observations on transference-love'. In *The Standard Edition of the Complete Psychological Works of Sigmund Freud. Vol. 12.*. London: Hogarth Press.

Freud, S. (1924e). 'The loss of reality in neurosis and psychosis'. In *The standard edition of the complete psychological works of Sigmund Freud. Vol. 19*. London: Hogarth Press.

Ironside, L. (1998). 'Serving two masters: a patient, a therapist, and an allegation of sexual abuse'. In V. Sinason (ed.), *Memory in Dispute* (pp. 95–120). London: Karnac Books.

Klein, M. (1946). 'Notes on some schizoid mechanisms'. In *The Writings of Melanie Klein, Vol. 3*. London: Hogarth. Reprinted in 1993. London: Karnac Books.

Mancia, M. (1993). 'Love and death in the transference: the case of the Hungarian poet Attila Jozsef'. *Psychoanalytic Psychotherapy*, 7(3), 253–264.

Milton, J. (1994). 'Abuser and abuse: Perverse solutions following childhood abuse'. *Psychoanalytic Psychotherapy*, 8(3), 243–255.

Putnam, F. (1985). 'Dissociation as a response to extreme trauma'. In R. Kluff (ed.), *Childhood Antecedents of Multiple Personality Disorder*. Washington, DC: American Psychiatric Press.

Reder, P. and Duncan, S. (1993). 'Closure, covert warnings and escalating child abuse'. *Child Abuse and Neglect*, 19(12), 1517–1521.

Rosenfeld, H. (1971). 'A clinical approach to the psychoanalytic theory of the life and death instincts'. *International Journal of Psychoanalysis*, 52.

Searle, J. (1969). *Speech Acts: An Essay in the Philosophy of Language*. New York: Cambridge University Press.

Segal, H. (1981). *The Work of Hannah Segal: A Kleinian Approach to Clinical Practice*. Northvale, NJ: Jason Aronson. Reprinted in 1988. London: Karnac Books.

Segal, H. (1991). *Dream, Phantasy and Art*. London: Routledge.

Sinason, M. (1993). 'Who is the mad voice inside?' *Psychoanalytic Psychotherapy*, 7(3), 207–221.

Sinason, V. (ed.) (1994). *Treating Survivors of Satanist Abuse*. London: Routledge.

Steiner, J. (1993). *Psychic Retreats: Pathological Organizations in Psychotic, Neurotic and Borderline Patients*. London: Routledge.

Stern, D. (1993). 'Acting versus remembering and transference love and infantile love'. In E. Person, A. Hagelin and P. Fonagy (eds.), *On Freud's 'Observations on Transference-Love'* (pp. 172–159). London: Karnac Books.

Szur, R. and Miller, S. (1992). *Extending Horizons: Psychoanalytic Psychotherapy with Children, Adolescents and Families*. London: Karnac Books.

Winnicott, D. W. (1960a). *The Maturational Processes and the Facilitating Environment*. Routledge. Reprinted London: Karnac Books, 1990.

Winnicott, D. W. (1960b). 'The theory of the parent-infant relationship'. *International Journal of Psycho-Analysis*, 41, 585–595.

Chapter 9

Armstrong, D. (2005). *Organization in the Mind: Psychoanalysis, Group Relations, and Organizational Consultancy*. London: H. Karnac (Books) Ltd.

Bion, W. R. (1962a). *Learning from Experience*. London: Karnac Books.

Brenman Pick, I. (1985). 'Working through in the countertransference'. *International Journal of Psychoanalysis*, 66, 157–166.

Carpy, D. V. (1989). 'Tolerating the countertransference: a mutative process'. *The International Journal of Psychoanalysis*, 70, 287–294.

Casement, P. (1985). *On Learning from the Patient*. London: Routledge.

Freud, S. (1912e). 'Recommendations to physicians practising psycho-analysis'. *The standard edition of the complete psychological works of Sigmund Freud. Vol. 12* (pp. 109–120). London: Hogarth Press.

Freud, S. (1915e). 'The unconscious'. *The Standard Edition of the Complete Psychological Works of Sigmund Freud*, Vol. 14 (pp. 159–215). London: Hogarth Press.

Gabbard, G. O. (1995). 'The early history of boundary violations in psychoanalysis'. *Journal of the American Psychoanalytic Association*, 43(4), 1115–1136.

Gabbard, G. (2000). 'Disguise or consent: problems and recommendations concerning the publication and presentation of clinical material'. *Journal of the American Psychoanalytic Association*, 81, 1071–1086 (Ethics).

Jaques, E. (1951). *The Changing Culture of a Factory: A Study of Authority and Participation in an Industrial Setting*. London: Routledge & Kegan Paul Ltd.

Stapley, L. F. (1996). *The Personality of the Organization: A Psycho-dynamic Explanation of Culture and Change*. London: Free Association Books.

Stokoe, P. (2020). *The Curiosity Drive: Our Need for Inquisitive Thinking*. Bicester: Phoenix Publishing House.

Chapter 10

Dineen, M. (2002). *Six Steps to Root Cause Analysis*. Oxford: Consequence.

Horsfall, S. (2014). 'Doctors who commit suicide while under GMC fitness to practise investigation'. General Medical Council. www.gmc-uk.org/-/media/documents/Internal_review_into_suicide_in_FTP_processes.pdf_59088696.pdf (Accessed 7 July 2022).

Chapter 11

Barlow, D. (2010). 'Negative effects from psychological treatments: A perspective'. *American Psychologist*, 65(1), 13–20. DOI: 10.1037/a0015643.

Bowlby Centre (2021). *The Bowlby Centre complaints procedure*. https://the bowlbycentre.org.uk/members-area/complaints-procedure (Accessed 3 September 2021).

British Association for Counselling and Psychotherapy (2021a). *Public Protection Committee: 2020 annual report*. www.bacp.co.uk/media/11019/bacp-ppc-annual-report-2020.pdf (Accessed 2 September 2021).

British Association for Counselling and Psychotherapy. (2021b). *Members taking part in protests*. Rugby: BACP. www.bacp.co.uk/membership/membership-policies/ (Accessed 12 September 2021).

British Psychological Society. (2020). *Minutes of the Board of Trustees meeting in December*

2020. www.bps.org.uk/system/files/Secure%20-%20Member%20and% 20Subscriber/Board%20of%20Trustees%20Minutes%20-%20December%202020.pdf (Accessed 2 September 2021; member log in required).

Cambridge Dictionary. (2021a). 'Definition of misuse'. https://dictionary.cambridge.org/dictionary/english/misuse (Accessed 1 September 2021).

Cambridge Dictionary. (2021b). 'Definition of abuse'. Available at: https://dictionary.cambridge.org/dictionary/english/abuse (Accessed 1 September 2021).

Clark, D. (2016). 'The improving access to psychological therapies (IAPT) programme: Background, strengths, weaknesses and future direction'. Keynote, Division of Counselling Psychology Annual Conference, 8 July 2016. Brighton, UK.

Cox, P. K. (2017a). *Opening up Pandora's box: Unintended harm in the consultation room*. Doctoral dissertation, University of Surrey, Guildford, England. http://epubs.surrey.ac.uk/844835/ (Accessed 4 September 2021).

Cox, P. K. (2017b). 'Informed consent: Legal changes, dilemmas and complaints'. https://theprofessionalpractitioner.net/2017/10/23/article-june-1st-2021 (Accessed 8 July 2022).

Cox, P. K. (2018). 'Naming and shaming therapists: Protecting the public or harming therapy?' Presentation to the Psychologists Protection Society, 3 November 2018, Manchester, England. https://theprofessionalpractitioner.net/cpd-activities/ (Accessed 8 July 2022).

Cox, P. (2019). 'The psychological impacts of racial discrimination for both clients and practitioners in complaints procedures and professional conduct hearings'. Presentation at the BPS (Black and Asian Therapy Group), conference *Psychological impacts of racial discrimination for both clients and practitioners*, 11 October 2019, De Vere Grand Connaught Rooms, London.

Cox, P. (2020). 'Complaints and minority health care professionals – How far do disciplinary procedures reflect wider social discriminations?' Online presentation to NHS Complex Trauma Service – Berkshire Traumatic Stress Service, 15 October 2020.

Cox, P. (2021). 'The HCPC should support climate change activists, not question their fitness to practise'. *Clinical Psychology Forum Special Issue: Climate Change*, 346, 35–41.

Cox, P. K. and Shohet, R. (2017). 'Mapping transferences in complaints procedures: The shadow of therapeutic work'. *CSTD Annual Conference. Exploring the Dynamics of Complaints: From Complaints to Commitment*. Centre for Supervision and Team Development, 6 July 2017, London.

Fleischer, J. A. and Wissler, A. (1985). 'The therapist as patient: Special problems and considerations'. *Psychotherapy: Theory, Research, Practice, Training*, 22(3), 587–594. DOI: 10.1037/h0085544.

Fonagy, P. (2012). 'Tavistock Adult Depression Study (TADS): A randomised controlled trial of psychoanalytic psychotherapy for treatment-resistant/treatment-refractory forms of depression'. Presentation of findings, London: University College, 11 March 2012.

Gillick v West Norfolk and Wisbech Area Health Authority and Department of Health and Social Security. (1984). QBD 581. As cited in 'Children's Legal Centre (1985) Landmark decision for children's rights', *Childright*, 22, 11–18.

Glyde, T. (2016). 'Sex work – society's transactional blind spot'. *The Lancet Psychiatry*, 3(7), 614–615. DOI: 10.1016/S2215-0366(16)30126-2.

Hallam, R. (2019). *Common Sense for the 21st Century: Only nonviolent rebellion can now stop climate breakdown and social collapse*. London: Chelsea Green Publishing.

Health and Care Professions Council (2015). *The costs of fitness to practise: a study of the Health and Care Professions Council*. www.hcpc-uk.org/globalassets/resources/reports/research/the-costs-of-fitness-to-practise---a-study-of-the-health-and-care-professions-council.pdf (Accessed 13 September 2021).

Health and Care Professions Council (2018). Council meeting, 19 September 2018. www.hcpc-uk.org/news-and-events/meetings/2018/september/

council-meeting---19-september-2018/. (Accessed 12 September 2021).

Health and Care Professions Council. (2019). 'Threshold policy for fitness to practise investigations'. www.hcpc-uk.org/resources/policy/threshold-policy-for-fitness-to-practise-investigations/ (Accessed 2 September 2021).

Health and Care Professions Council. (2020). 'Protecting the public: Promoting professionalism 1 April 2018 to 31 March 2019'. *Fitness to practise annual report 2019*. London: HCPC. www.hcpc-uk.org/registrants/updates/2020/what-our-fitness-to-practise-annual-report-shows (Accessed 15 August 2021).

Health and Care Professions Council. (2021). *Standards of conduct, performance and ethics*. London: HCPC. www.hcpc-uk.org/standards/standards-of-conduct-performance-and-ethics (Accessed 23 September 2021).

Health and Safety Executive. (2021). *Discontinuing a prosecution*. www.hse.gov.uk/enforce/enforcementguide/court/magistrates-discontinue.htm (Accessed 31 August 2021).

House, R. (2008). 'Training and education for therapeutic practitionership: "Tranmodern" perspectives'. *Counselling Psychology Quarterly*, 21(1), 1–10. DOI: 10.1080/09515070801899867.

Hyde, J. (2021). 'SRA ordered to pay £27,000 over "heavy handed" tribunal pursuit, *The Law Gazette*. www.lawgazette.co.uk/news/sra-ordered-to-pay-27000-over-heavy-handed-tribunal-pursuit/5106877.article. (Accessed 31 August 2021).

Jacobs, M. (2001). 'Some underlying psychodynamics of complaint'. In R. Casemore (ed.), *Surviving complaints against counsellors and psychotherapists: Towards understanding and healing* (pp. 41–50). Ross-on-Wye: PCCS Books.

Jones, C. (2001). 'Acceptance of uncertainty'. In R. Casemore (ed.), *Surviving complaints against counsellors and psychotherapists: Towards understanding and healing* (pp. 131–142). Ross-on-Wye: PCCS Books.

Jones, R. (2020). 'I took my turn on Friday to be arrested'. *The Psychologist*, 33, 28–32. https://thepsychologist.bps.org.uk/volume-33/december-2020/i-took-my-turn-friday-be-arrested.

Kearns, K. (2011). *The mirror crack'd: When good enough therapy goes wrong and other cautionary tales for the humanistic practitioner*. London: Routledge.

Klein, M. (1946). 'Notes on some schizoid mechanisms'. *International Journal of Psycho-Analysis*, 27, 99–110.

Merton, R. K. (1936). 'The unanticipated consequences of purposeful social action'. *American Sociological Review*, 1(6), 894–904. DOI: 10.2307/2084615.

Merton, R. K. (1972). 'Insiders and outsiders: A chapter in the sociology of knowledge'. In 'Varieties of political expression in sociology', *American Journal of Sociology*, 78(1), 9–47. www.jstor.org/stable/2776569 (Accessed 8 July 2022).

National Counselling Society (2020). *Code of ethical practice*. https://nationalcounsellingsociety.org/assets/uploads/docs/cs/National-Counselling-Society-Code-of-Ethics.pdf (Accessed 13 September 2021).

Professional Standards Authority (2016). *Regulation rethought: Proposal for reform*. London: PSA. www.professionalstandards.org.uk/docs/default-source/publications/thought-paper/regulation-rethought.pdf?sfvrsn=c537120_20. (Accessed 31 August 2021).

Professional Standards Authority (2020). *Annual review of accreditation 2019/20 National Counselling Society (NCS) and National Hypnotherapy Society (HS) December 2020*. www.professionalstandards.org.uk/docs/default-source/accredited-registers/panel-decisions/annual-review-panel-decision-ncs-hs.pdf?sfvrsn=33297f 20_ 12 (Accessed 2 September 2021).

Professional Standards Authority (2021a). *Annual review of accreditation 2020/21 British Psychoanalytic Council (BPC) February 2021*.

Professional Standards Authority (2021b). *Annual review of accreditation 2019/20 United Kingdom Council for Psychotherapy (UKCP) January 2021*.

Professional Standards Authority. (2021c). *Performance review 2020/21: Health and Care Professions Council.* London: PSA. performance-review-hcpc-2020-21.pdf (Accessed 12 September 2021).

Shohet, R. (2017). 'Exploring the dynamics of complaints'. *Self & Society*, 45(1), 69–71. DOI: 10.1080/03060497.2017.1290452.

Social Care. (2020). *Types and indicators of abuse.* www.scie.org.uk/safeguarding/adults/introduction/types-and-indicators-of-abuse#psychological. (Accessed 1 September 2021).

Strupp, H. H., Hadley, S. W. and Gomes-Schwartz, B. (1977). *Psychotherapy for better or worse.* New York: Jason Aronson, Inc. DOI:10.1192/S0007125000004359.

Totton, N. (2001). 'Scapegoats and sacred cows: Towards good enough conflict resolution'. In R. Casemore (ed.), *Surviving complaints against counsellors and psychotherapists: Towards understanding and healing* (pp. 99–109). Ross-on-Wye: PCCS Books.

United Kingdom Council for Psychotherapy (2021). *UKCP position statement: Protests.* London: UKCP: www.psychotherapy.org.uk/news/ukcp-position-statement-protests/ (Accessed 25 August 2021).

Williams, F., Coyle, A. and Lyons, E. (1999). 'How counselling psychologists view their personal therapy'. *The British Journal of Medical Psychology*, 27(3), 545–555. DOI: 10.1348/000711299160112.

Winnicott, D. (1947). *Through paediatrics to psychoanalysis.* Collected Papers: London.

Van der Kolk, B. (2014). *The body keeps the score.* London: Penguin.

Chapter 12

Bowlby Centre (2021). *The Bowlby Centre complaints procedure.* https://the bowlbycentre.org.uk/members-area/complaints-procedure (Accessed 3 September 2021).

British Association of Counsellors and Psychotherapists (2018). *Ethical framework for the counselling professions.* Rugby: BACP. www.bacp.co.uk/events-and-resources/ethics-and-standards/ethical-framework-for-the-counselling-professions/ (Accessed 5 September 2021).

British Medical Association. (2021). *GMC investigation support – Doctor support service.* www.bma.org.uk/advice-and-support/your-wellbeing/wellbeing-support-services/gmc-investigation-support-doctor-support-service (Accessed 8 July 2022).

British Psychoanalytic Council. (2011). *Code of ethics.* London: BPC. www.bpc.org.uk/download/745/4.1-Code-of-Ethics-Feb-2011-no-numbers.pdf. (Accessed 6 September 2021).

Care Quality Commission. (2021). *Updated guidance on meeting the duty of candour.* Published/posted [online] 11 March 2021. www.cqc.org.uk/news/stories/updated-guidance-meeting-duty-candour (Accessed 9 September 2021).

Cox, P. K. (2017). *Opening up Pandora's box: Unintended harm in the consultation room.* Doctoral dissertation, University of Surrey, Guildford, England. http://epubs.surrey.ac.uk/844835/ (Accessed 3 September 2021).

Cox, P. K. (2018). 'Naming and shaming therapists: Protecting the public or harming therapy?' Presentation to the Psychologists Protection Society, 3 November 2018, Manchester, England. https://theprofessionalpractitioner.net/cpd-activities/ (Accessed 8 July 2022).

Cox, P. (2019). 'The psychological impacts of racial discrimination for both clients and practitioners in complaints procedures and professional conduct hearings'. Presentation at the BPS (Black and Asian Therapy Group), conference *Psychological impacts of racial discrimination for both clients and practitioners*, 11 October 2019, De Vere Grand Connaught Rooms, London.

Cox, P. (2021). 'The HCPC should support climate change activists, not question their fitness to practise'. *Clinical Psychology Forum Special Issue: Climate Change*, 346, 35–41.

Cox, P. and, Aella. (2020). 'Whore phobia: The experiences of a dual-training sex worker–psychotherapist'. *Psychotherapy and Politics International*, 18(2), e1539. DOI: 10.1002/ppi.1539.

Health and Care Professions Council. (2019). 'Threshold policy for fitness to practise investigations'. www.hcpc-uk.org/resources/policy/threshold-policy-for-fitness-to-practise-investigations/ (Accessed 2 September 2021).

Hewitt, W. (2020a). *Professional Standards Authority for Health & Social Care v Health and Care Professions Council & R* [2020] 3 WLUK 95

Hewitt, W. (2020b). *Wendy Hewitt successfully defends paramedic in High Court appeal brought by the PSA*. London: 5SAH. www.5sah.co.uk/knowledge-hub/news/2020-03-11/wendy-hewitt-successfully-defends-paramedic-in-high-court-appeal-brought-by-the-psa (Accessed 3 September 2021).

House of Commons (2019). *Counsellors and Psychotherapists (Regulation) and Conversion Therapy Bill 2017–19*. Posted 18 March, 2019. https://services.Parliament.uk/Bills/2017-19/counsellorsandpsychotherapistsregulationandconversiontherapy.html. (Accessed 10 September 2021).

Jones, S. (2016). *Talking therapists – what does the Statement of Intent mean for practitioners?* Kingsley Napley solicitors. Posted 5 January 2016. www.kingsleynapley.co.uk/insights/blogs/regulatory-blog/talking-therapists-what-does-the-statement-of-intent-mean-for-practitioners. (Accessed 16 September 2021).

Jones, S. and Norris, J. (2016). *'Dogged and obstinate' BACP prevented from proceeding to adjudicate on a complaint already disposed of by the UKCP*. Kingsley Napley solicitors. Posted 16 December 2016. www.kingsleynapley.co.uk/insights/blogs/regulatory-blog/dogged-and-obstinate-bacp-prevented-from-proceeding-to-adjudicate-on-a-complaint-already-disposed-of-by-the-ukcp. (Accessed 16 September 2021).

Karpman, S. B. (2014). *A game free life*. San Francisco: Drama Triangle Publications.

Mowbray, R. (1995). *The case against psychotherapy registration: A conservation issue for the human potential movement*. London: Trans Marginal Press.

Music, G. (2011). *Nurturing natures*. Hove: Psychology Press.

Norris, J. (2015). *Kingsley Napley force a consultation on new procedural rules for psychoanalysts*. Posted 5 January 2015. www.kingsleynapley.co.uk/insights/news/kingsley-napley-force-a-consultation-on-new-procedural-rules-for-psychoanalysts. (Accessed 3 September 2021).

Nursing and Midwifery Council. (2021). *New strategic direction: Ensuring public safety, enabling professionalism*. London: Nursing and Midwifery Council.

Palmer Barnes, F. (1998). *Complaints and grievances in psychotherapy: A handbook of ethical practice*. London: Routledge.

Pink Therapy (2017). *Memorandum of understanding on Conversion Therapy in the UK: Version 2*. https://pinktherapyblog.com/tag/memorandum-of-understanding. (Accessed 9 September 2021).

Postle, D. and House, R. (eds) (2009). *Compliance? Ambivalence? Rejection? Nine papers challenging the Health Professions Council July 2009 proposals for the state regulation of the psychological therapies*. WLR/eIpnosis Production for the Alliance for Counselling and Psychotherapy Against State Regulation, supported by the Independent Practitioners Network. https://allianceblogs.files.wordpress.com/2014/05/complianceambivalencerejection2009.pdf (Accessed 8 July 2022)

Professional Standards Authority (2016). *Regulation rethought: Proposal for reform*. London: PSA.

Professional Standards Authority (2019a). *Annual review of accreditation 2019/20 British Psychoanalytic Council (BPC) December 2019*. London: PSA. www.

professionalstandards.org.uk/what-we-do/accredited-registers/find-a-register/detail/british-psychoanalytic-council (Accessed 8 July 2022).

Professional Standards Authority (2019b). *Annual review of accreditation 2019/20 UK Council for Psychotherapy (UKCP) November 2019*. London: PSA. www.professionalstandards.org.uk/what-we-do/accredited-registers/find-a-register/detail/uk-council-for-psychotherapy (Accessed 8 July 2022).

Professional Standards Authority (2020a). *Annual review of accreditation 2019/20 British Association for Counselling and Psychotherapy (BACP) August 2020*. London: PSA.

Professional Standards Authority (2020b). *Performance Review 2019/20: Health and Care Professions Council*. London: PSA. www.professional standards.org.uk/docs/default-source/publications/performance-reviews/performance-review-hcpc-2019-20.pdf?sfvrsn=630a7620_5. (Accessed 9 September 2021).

Professional Standards Authority (2020c). *Consultation on the future shape of the Accredited Registers programme*. www.professionalstandards.org.uk/what-we-do/improving-regulation/consultation/consultation-on-future-of-accredited-registers (Accessed 8 July 2022).

Professional Standards Authority (2021a). *Annual review of accreditation 2020/21 British Psychoanalytic Council (BPC)*. London: PSA. www.professionalstandards.org.uk/what-we-do/accredited-registers/find-a-register/detail/british-psychoanalytic-council (Accessed 8 July 2022).

Professional Standards Authority (2021b). *Annual review of accreditation 2020/21 UK Council for Psychotherapy (UKCP) January 2021*. London: PSA. www.professionalstandards.org.uk/what-we-do/accredited-registers/find-a-register/detail/uk-council-for-psychotherapy (Accessed 8 July 2022).

Professional Standards Authority (2021c). *Annual review of accreditation 2020/2021 British Association for Counselling and Psychotherapy (BACP) August 2021*. London: PSA. www.professionalstandards.org.uk/docs/default-source/accredited-registers/panel-decisions/bacp-annual-review-2021.pdf?sfvrsn=84357220_12 (Accessed 8 July 2022)

Professional Standards Authority (2021d). *Performance Review 2020/21: Health and Care Professions Council. London: PSA*. www.professionalstandards.org.uk/docs/default-source/publications/performance-reviews/performance-review-hcpc-2019-20.pdf?sfvrsn=630a7620_5 (Accessed 8 July 2022).

Psychotherapy and Counselling Union (2017). *Training and employment code of practice*. www.psychotherapyandcounsellingunion.co.uk/codes-of-practice (Accessed 8 July 2022).

Psychotherapy and Counselling Union (2021). *Who we are*. www.psychotherapyandcounsellingunion.co.uk/ (Accessed 3 September 2021).

Psychotherapists and Counsellors for Social Responsibility (2015). *Changing the game*. Psychotherapists and Counsellors for Social Responsibility conference at the Resource Centre, 5 September, 2015, London, UK.

Rowland, A. (2017). 'GMC fitness to practise procedures: Interview with Anna Rowland'. *Medical Doctors Union Journal*, Autumn (Online), 6-10. https://mdujournal.themdu.com/issue-archive/autumn-2017/gmc-fitness-to-practise-procedures (Accessed 10 September 2021).

Stern, D. (2000). *The interpersonal world of the infant*. London: Basic Books.

Shohet, R. (2017). 'Exploring the dynamics of complaints'. *Self & Society*, 45(1), 69–71. DOI: 10.1080/03060497.2017.1290452.

Totton, N. (2000). 'Beyond complaint: Client-practitioner conflict and the Independent Practitioners Network'. *Self & Society*, 45(1), 69–71. DOI: 10.1080/03060497.2000.11086005.

Totton, N. (2001). 'Scapegoats and sacred cows: Towards good enough conflict resolution'. In R. Casemore (ed.), *Surviving complaints against counsellors and psychotherapists:*

Towards understanding and healing (pp. 99–109). Ross-on-Wye: PCCS Books.

UNISON (2021). *HCPC registration fee rise*. Available at: www.unison.org.uk/health-news/2021/02/hcpc-registration-fee-rise (Accessed 14 September 2021).

United Kingdom Council for Psychotherapy. (2012). *UKCP's complaints and conduct process*. www.psychotherapy.org.uk/ukcp-members/complaints/how-to-make-a-complaint (Accessed 8 July 2022).

United Kingdom Council for Psychotherapy. (2019). *Code of ethics and professional practice*. www.psychotherapy.org.uk/media/v11peyoh/ukcp-code-of-ethics-and-professional-practice-2019.pdf (Accessed 3 September 2021).

Van der Kolk, B. (2014). *The body keeps the score*. London: Penguin.

Wampold, B. E., and Imel, Z. E. (2015). *The great psychotherapy debate: The evidence for what makes psychotherapy work*. 2nd edn. New York: Routledge.

Chapter 13

Association of Child Psychotherapists (ACP), (2017) *Code of Professional Conduct*. https://childpsychotherapy.org.uk/search (Accessed 8 July 2022).

Association of Child Psychotherapists (ACP), (2019). *Disciplinary Procedure*. https://childpsychotherapy.org.uk/acp-register-standards/standards-practice/disciplinary-procedure (Accessed 8 July 2022) updated March 2021.

British Association for Counselling & Psychotherapy (BACP), (2018). *Professional Conduct Procedure*. www.bacp.co.uk/about-us/protecting-the-public/professional-conduct/professional-conduct-procedure (Accessed 8 July 2022).

British Psychoanalytic Council (BPC), (2016). *Complaints Procedure*. www.bpc.org.uk/download/2276/Complaints-Procedure-Amended-01.21.pdf (Accessed 8 July 2022).

UK Council for Psychotherapy (UKCP), (2017). *Complaints and Conduct Process*. www.psychotherapy.org.uk/ukcp-members/complaints/how-to-make-a-complaint (Accessed 8 July 2022).

UK Council for Psychotherapy (UKCP), (2019). *Code of Ethics and Professional Practice*. www.psychotherapy.org.uk/media/v11peyoh/ukcp-code-of-ethics-and-professional-practice-2019.pdf (Accessed 8 July 2022).

INDEX

Karnac Books, founded in 1950 and relaunched in 2020, publishes seminal and contemporary texts on psychotherapy and psychoanalysis. It continues its long tradition of exploring the intricacies of these disciplines, providing space for the best writers on the complexities of the mind.